Keto-Reset Cookbook

Reboot Your Metabolism With Delicious Ketogenic Recipes And Burn Fat Forever

Table of Contents

What is the Keto Reset? **6**

What does it mean to reboot your metabolism? 7

How to burn fat with Ketogenic diet recipes 11

Allowable Foods & Non-Allowable Foods............................16

Ketogenic Diet Recipes **22**

  Breakfast **23**

    Cauliflower Hash Browns with Onions and Chives 23

    Breakfast Bagels.. 24

    Baked Bacon Omelet 26

    Poached Eggs in Spiced Tomato Sauce 27

    Brussels Sprouts and Eggs Hash 28

    Shrimp Omelet.. 29

    Hash Browns / Spaghetti Squash 30

    Turkey Breakfast Wrap..31

    Sausage Breakfast Sandwich 32

    Cauliflower Hash Brown Waffles 33

    No-Crust Spinach Quiche 34

    Salmon Breakfast Balls 35

    Breakfast Salad 37

    Chorizo Sausage, Goat Cheese, Spinach Omelet............38

  Meat **39**

    Salisbury Steak.. 39

    Zucchini Beef Stir Fry 40

    Keto Cabbage Casserole..41

    Crispy Pork Bites 42

    Meat Stuffed Zucchini Boats 43

    Keto Beef Stroganoff.. 44

    Jalapeno Cheddar Beef or Turkey Burgers 45

    Crock Pot Pulled Pork.. 46

    Eggplant N Beef Pizza 47

    Bacon-Cheeseburger Casserole 48

    Beef 'N "Rice"... 49

    Beef and Zucchini Burgers..50

Poultry **51**
Lettuce Wraps with Chicken Salad 51
Chicken Casserole 52
Keto Chicken Pad Thai 53
Quick 'N Easy Buffalo Wings 54
Chicken Curry 55
Chicken Stew – Crockpot Style 56
Chicken Enchilada Keto-Style 57
Easy Lemon Fried Chicken 58
Spinach-Stuffed Chicken 59
Chicken Kiev 60
Chicken Chili 61
Creamy Tuscan Chicken 62
Bacon-Ranch Chicken Casserole 63
Leftover Turkey (or Chicken) Casserole 64
Chicken Pot Pie 65
Chicken "n Cream with Poblano Peppers 67
Turkey Meatballs and Kale Soup 68
Chicken Zucchini Pasta with Pistachios 70
Seafood **72**
Pan-Roasted Salmon with Red Cabbage 72
Watercress & Herb Sauce with Fish 73
Fish Chowder 74
Halibut with Parmesan Crust 75
Lemon-Garlic Shrimp 76
Creamy Fish Casserole 77
Salmon/Avocado Salsa 78
Tuna Fish Patties 79
Salmon Cucumber Wraps 80
Quick 'n Easy Shrimp Scampi 81
Keto Fish Nuggets 82
Spicy Fish Stew 83
One-Pan Lemon, Butter, Garlic Shrimp with Asparagus 84
Shrimp and Sausage Skillet 86
Wasabi Salmon Burgers 87
Appetizer **88**
Cheddar Cheese Chips and Bacon Guacamole 88
Low Carb Caprese Meatballs 89
Frittata and Tomatoes 90

Deviled Eggs with Avocado 91
Cauliflower Grilled Cheese 92
Greek Avocado Salad 93
Onion Soup 94
Cucumber Bites 95
Grilled Tomatoes and Apricot Jam 96
Fried Green Beans 97
Kale Chips 98
Coconut Chocolate Bars 99
Deviled Eggs with Bacon 100
Twice Baked "potato" Zucchini 101
Snack 102
Roasted Garlic Spinach and Bacon Dip 102
Mini Cheesecakes 103
Freezer Fudge 104
Zucchini Chips 105
Fat Bomb! 106
Coconut Berry Drops 107
Lime Popsicles 108
Veggie Dip (A lot like hummus!) 109
White chocolate Butter Pecan Fat Bomb 110
Chocolate Mousse 111
Keto Smoothie 112
Loaded Hassel back (not potatoes but) Zucchini 113
Fast and Easy Blueberry Smoothie 114
Mexican Chocolate Pudding 115
Conclusion 116

What is the Keto Reset?

Perhaps you've heard a little about the Keto diet, or the Keto reset and wondered how it works. The Keto diet is a lifestyle in which you eat less carbs, less protein and higher amounts of fat. The reasoning behind this eating plan is to reset the body. The human liver produces ketones that the body uses for energy. When you consume high carbohydrate foods, the body produces more insulin and glucose in response. The body easily converts glucose molecules to energy. Since glucose molecules are small and easy to convert, they are the first choice for a source of energy. Insulin is then produced to help carry glucose throughout the body.

Your body prefers to use glucose as a primary energy source, which leaves fats sitting there, unused. They are treated as a sort of reserve supply. The end result is pockets of stored fat of excess weight. For most people, their diet includes large amounts of carbs. Carbohydrates, though are changed to sugar or glucose, which means the body uses it for energy. By greatly reducing the amount of carbs you eat, you send your body into a state of *ketosis*. This is a natural process initiated by the body to help with survival when you're not eating enough food. It's important to note that there is a difference between your body going into a healthy state of ketosis where it starts using stored fat for energy and going into starvation mode.

When the body goes into ketosis, it produces ketones. These are produced during the process of the liver breaking down fats. The goal of the Keto diet is forcing the body into this type of metabolic state. It doesn't work by trying to starve ourselves, though. The body doesn't reset like that if we starve ourselves of calories alone. It will try to save as much "resources' as possible in starvation mode. This is counter-productive. But the reset occurs naturally if we starve the body of carbs specifically.

It's funny and amazing how our body adapts to what we feed it. It can be forced into a Keto reset if it's overloaded with fats and lacking in carbohydrates. That's when it starts to burn ketones as its primary energy source instead of the carbs it is used to turning into energy.

The Reset!

The definition of "Ketogenic" or being in the state of "Ketosis" simply means the body burned off all the sugars that were dumped in the bloodstream after eating carbs. Eating a Keto diet, resets the body by forcing it to switch over from burning carbs to use for energy to burn stored fat for fuel. The reset takes place in the liver as it aids the body in the digestive process. Webster's Dictionary defines ketosis as an increase of ketone bodies throughout the body when carbohydrate intake is reduced and the rate of carbohydrate metabolism slows. Ketones are produced by a higher consumption of fat, increasing the body's metabolism. When your body is releasing ketones, it is in ketosis. Consuming less carbs means there are less for the body to metabolize and use for energy. This shifts, or resets, the body and increases its fat-burning potential which causes the loss of extra weight.

Benefits of a Keto Reset and Ketogenic Diet

Years ago, when researchers started studying low carb dieting, the primary interest was not for weight loss, even though this is one of the primary benefits. Professionals in the medical field, including scientists and doctors, were interested in being able to manage health problems by controlling the diet. What they discovered was that the Keto reset was indeed useful for losing weight, but also had many other health benefits. Many were quite surprised at the improvement in the way they feel above the weight loss they achieve.

What does it mean to reboot your metabolism?

Obtaining the state of ketosis can help change metabolism. Remember, normally, the body breaks down carbs into glucose, so it can be used to energize the body. Most people look at carbohydrates as the dietary way to provide fuel for the body. But when the body is fed a Ketogenic diet, it reaches the state of ketosis. Now the body metabolizes fats changing them into ketone bodies to use for energy. Ketones provide a constant source of energy for the body instead of intermittently like carbs. When your body reaches ketosis, your metabolism literally shifts, or reboots. Ketosis can be a powerful way to maintain a healthy metabolism.

Why can't I just count calories?

Counting calories and reducing the number of calories you consume is not an effective way to reboot your metabolism. As a matter of fact, it is quite the opposite and you can wind up losing muscle tone should your body think it's starving. We're talking about two different metabolic responses here. When you reduce your caloric intake, you send signals to your body that there's not enough food to go around. It starts storing fat to prevent starvation. But the Keto reset will inform the body that it's all good now. Your metabolism isn't shifted into preventing starvation mode. Instead your body starts consuming fat instead of storing it. If you just reduce caloric intake, your metabolism dips, your weight loss plateaus and then you regain any weight you may have lost as a result. But when you boost your metabolism and your body is in a state of ketosis, the metabolic response differs. The three things that happens in response are:

- Increase in growth hormones to help retain muscle mass
- Insulin drops and prevents insulin resistance
- Hormone levels of norepinephrine increase and keeps your basal metabolism boosted

How does the metabolism benefit from ketosis?

The body burns off the glycogen it makes from the carbs you eat. At this point, your body will start burning through its own fat storage. This is what is meant by ketosis. This state occurs when you eat a Ketogenic diet. Once the body starts burning through stored fat, it will maintain a healthy metabolism because energy is available to be burned. When you simply "diet" the metabolism slows down, but in a state of ketosis, metabolism gets a boost. There are several benefits you'll realize when your metabolism switches over from burning carbs to using fatty acids for energy. These include:

- More burning of fat
- Reduced inflammation
- Longer, fuller life
- Improved immunity
- Brain protection
- Lower risk of cancer
- Clearer thinking

Many times, the problems people have with their metabolism are related to the body not responding properly to insulin. This is a substance released by the body in response to glucose entering the bloodstream. If a person's glucose levels are too high, then they can become insulin resistant. For many people this leads to diabetes or numerous other health problems. When you constantly consume high carb foods, your insulin levels keep spiking. This can lead to various issues with a person's metabolism. A Ketogenic diet which restricts carbohydrate intake is often very effective at helping maintain healthy insulin levels.

How does ketosis or low-carb intake affect metabolism?

Ketosis brings about a metabolic change, and this is different than what benefits there may be to simply eating a low-carb diet. The Keto diet is sometimes just considered "low carb" but it's much more than that as it facilitates a metabolic change by converting fats into energy. There are a few benefits in eating a lower carbohydrate diet, but you'll realize a lot more once the body goes into ketosis. You may feel tired and weak if you just cut out carbs, but ketosis will help the body efficiently burn fats and doesn't have any ill, long-term side effects. When just cutting out carbs you may encounter:

- Hunger pangs
- Hormonal disruption
- Moodiness
- Irritableness
- Unexpected weight gain
- Decreased physical performance

If you just eat low carb and your body is not in a state of ketosis, the body still tries to use carbs and proteins for energy. It's looking for a fuel source that it's not being given. That won't help your metabolism or your mood.

How to measure your metabolism when in ketosis?

Earlier, how to know if you are in ketosis was discussed. How do you know then, how ketosis is improving your metabolism? There are two measurements that can be used to determine if ketosis is working on behalf of your metabolic heath.

Metabolism and Glucose Ketone Index

Over the last few years there has been much research and study about the glucose ketone index ratio, and how it is related to a person's metabolic health. The GKI is a good way to monitor how ketosis is affecting your metabolism and other body functions. The GKI is a ratio that is calculated by using your ketone level and glucose level. Divide your glucose level by your ketone level. This number is your metabolic state. Knowing and tracking the GKI can be a large part of preventing diabetes, obesity, cancer and other serious metabolic conditions. Studies have shown maintaining a low or moderate ketosis can help prevent many diseases and higher levels of ketosis can be a powerful tool with even more benefits such as helping to fight cancer.

Testing Ketones

There are three different ketones in the body, beta-hydroxybutyrate, acetone and acetoacetate. Each compound does different things when it comes to the metabolism of ketosis, and different ways to measure them. Some forms of measuring are better than others for different reasons. The three ketones are measurable as they move into different areas of the body, urine, blood and breath. These can be tested at home without requiring lab, technicians or expensive equipment. Taking these different measurements can be useful in determining how your body reacts to different variables. how the body reacts to exercise, and different types or amounts of foods. It is important to note that the optimal ketone level can be very individual. Knowing the numbers where you thrive along with the goal you are aiming at is a faster way to reach them, as long as you consistently check your numbers to make sure you are staying in your range.

Testing Acetoacetate Using Urine Strips

Excessive levels of acetoacetate can be detected in the urine. These ketones are only present in the urine if there is an excessive amount of them in the body. Once they are in excess, they can spill over into the urine. However, this is a good thing. As carbs increase in the blood stream and become abundant, the body secretes insulin in response and to help convert the carbs to fat. As ketones increase, rather than being stored as fat, they are excreted through the urine. Once your body starts producing ketones, they aren't all used up which means you can use a simple urine strip to see if your body is getting rid of the excess. When the urine has a high level of acetoacetate particularly, the strip will change color.

Please note that this test alone is not always reliable. As the body changes and adapts to ketosis, it will become more efficient at using the extra acetoacetate and ketone levels will be lower. This can be misleading since you are in a deeper state of ketosis despite what the stirp says. Hydration levels can also affect the strip reading. With these caveats, the advantage is still that strips are inexpensive and easy to do. It can be extremely useful when you are just starting a Ketogenic diet and desire to monitor the transition. They are not the most reliable as you continue in a state of ketosis.

Testing Beta-hydroxybutyrate with a Blood Meter

Your body will produce the ketone beta-hydroxybutyrate and you can take it in a supplement. Beta-hydroxybutyrate, or BHB, enters a cell and is converted into acetoacetone before it is converted to acetyl. This means that BHB remains mostly in the blood, as it is in route to the cells. This means the blood can be checked for BHB. It can be done at home in a way similar to when diabetics check their blood sugar. Simply, prick a finger and squeeze out a drop of blood so it falls on the stick. The meter will tell you how much BHB is in the blood. Unlike urine tests, the blood test is more reliable. This is due to the fact it doesn't become diluted and the ketone doesn't change due to factors such as hydration. It is a consistent and reliable way to measure ketone levels. The only thing about checking your levels with the blood is that some may have an aversion to pricking their finger to draw blood. The strips are a little more expensive and it can add up if you check your blood twice a day to monitor ketone levels.

Using Breath to Test Ketones

A breath meter can also help measure ketones. Sometimes it is useful to confirm a blood or urine test. It can also be useful for those who have an aversion to bodily fluids or drawing your own blood. Acetone is produced when beta-hydroxybutyrate is metabolized. Levels of acetate correlate to the amount of BHB in the blood. A ketonix device can measure the amount of acetone by simply breathing in it.

How to burn fat with Ketogenic diet recipes

The Ketogenic diet is a nutrition plan built on consuming few carbohydrates, some protein and lots of "good" fats. Basically, the eating plan retrains the body's metabolism so that it runs by using fats, or ketone bodies. Some studies have indicated eating a Ketogenic diet can improve muscle development, reduce inflammation and help with insulin sensitivity. The eating plan is constructed around consuming fats like grass-fed butter, avocados, coconut products, pasture-raised meats, extra virgin olive oil and nuts and seeds. It also includes some low-carb herbs, vegetables and fruits. Fat intake should be about 60 to 80% of the entire caloric intake.

Forming Ketones

Your body uses either glucose or ketone bodies as a source of energy. Glucose is a primary source of energy for most because they supply their body with lots of sugar, protein and starches that are all turned into blood sugar. A person can switch this primary energy source over to fat by fasting, or by eating a low-carb, high fat, moderate protein diet. Ketone bodies are a byproduct formed when fatty acids are converted into fuel. The liver oxidizes fatty acids to produce energy. Others are partially oxidized and form acetoacetate. This substance is converted to beta-hydroxybutyric acid. These are called ketone bodies.

Ketones are used by any tissues which contain mitochondria, this includes both the brain and muscles.

Any diet that simply reduces caloric intake can be catabolic, which means it causes muscle loss. This is simply due to consuming less energy which forces the body to use other tissue for energy. In addition, many dieters increase aerobic exercise which can lead to even more muscle breakdown. In this state, the brain can also absorb more protein to make more glucose to use as energy. This is called gluconeogenesis.

What makes ketosis different, then? First, the brain prefers ketones for energy rather than glucose. This is good – because it means the body isn't breaking down protein to create energy. It forces the body to use fat reserves – like your love handles to create energy. This is one of the biggest benefits to eating a low carb diet.

What's cool though is that the body actually prefers using ketones for energy. It can run about 70% more efficiently than it does when using glucose for its primary source of energy. If you think about our ancestors, they didn't have glucose, or sugar to use as an energy source. They were more likely gaining energy from eating the fat from a saber-tooth tiger, or a wooly mammoth.

How does all this work?

By following a Keto diet, you convince your body to sort of switch gears – to ketosis. It takes a break from burning sugar, basically because it's no longer there. The liver is a factory, and its job is to break fatty acids down into ketones. The brain remember, can't absorb fatty acids. However, it does absorb ketones. After the body starts producing ketones, it moves them to the brain. The brain will make the switch from burning glucose for energy and start depending on ketones instead.

How do I make it happen?

For most people, the process of getting into the state of ketosis doesn't take too long. Basically, you'll increase your high-fat intake and reduce your protein while also decreasing your intake of carbs. Ultimately, when you break it down, the percentages will look something like this:

- Most of your calories will be from fats – between 60 and 70% of your caloric intake
- Protein should be between 20 and 30% of your daily caloric consumption

- Carbs should be held to no more than 50 grams each day and make up around 5 to 10% of your calories for a day

Please note that these numbers can be different for each person. You must take into account your specific, personal factors like gender, level of activity, lean body mass and your height and weight.

Is there a way to help my body burn fat during ketosis?

There are some definite strategies for using Ketogenic diet recipes to help your body burn more fat. The whole premise behind the diet is to provide the body with insufficient carbs and make it use fat for energy rather than glucose. Maybe you've got a lot of questions about now. How many carbs should you eat each day? Is there a best time to eat carbs? Are some carbs better than others for helping burn fat? Each person's metabolic makeup is different, and you'll have to find the strategy that works for you. Here are a few strategies to help you achieve your maximum fat-burning goals.

- Depending on your metabolism, consume around 30 to 50 grams of carbohydrates every day. Some individuals find that a carb-cycling strategy helps them achieve their goals and keeps the body from thinking it's going into starvation mode. This means about every five days double your carb intake. For just two days eat 60 to 100 carbs. For some, this help prevent plateaus.

- Stack your carb intake around workouts. Try consuming half of your daily carbs before a workout and the other half of them afterwards. For some people, it works better to eat all their carbs just before a workout, and for others, it works better to consume them all after. Also, consuming the bulk of your carbs in the morning can help the body switch to ketosis during the day and help you burn more fat.

- Take Branch Chain Amino Acids (BCAAs) to help the body continue to burn fat instead of muscle. These are special amino acids that trigger muscle building. Muscle tissue metabolizes them directly. Since they act like an energy source, they prevent the body from using muscles for fuel. You might try taking 5g just before or right after a workout. You can take them between meals or every two to three hours depending on what works for you.

- Saturated fats can also provide the body an energy source. These fats, from coconuts, are also naturally thermo-genic. This means they help increase fat burning. Try taking a teaspoon before and after a workout. You may also try taking it every couple of hours during the day.

- Keep your resistance workouts to no longer than an hour. This helps control cortisol levels. Cortisol is a stress hormone that. It slows down the fat burning process and metabolizes muscles. It's produced in a fight or flight response situation. Once you've been working out for an hour, hormones that build muscle tissue drop drastically, and cortisol levels increase greatly. You want to train optimally, not just harder every time. Help your body burn more fat by holding weight training and resistance exercises to under an hour.

Common Mistakes People Make on the Keto Diet

Even though following the Keto reset plan is simple, there are a few mistakes people make. The two most common ones include:

- Eating too many carbs
- Eating too much protein

Remember that elevating the number of ketones in the blood is essential to making this eating program a success. It's important to balance out your intake of calories, protein and carbs to achieve the results you want. If you eat too many carbs, you may still lose weight, but you will lose muscle and that is not what needs to happen. Consuming lower amounts of carbohydrates is essential to make the Keto reset happen.

Eating protein is good in general, and it is understood that protein builds muscle. But eating too much protein can prohibit your body from making the switch over to using fat for energy instead of carbs and end up deteriorating muscle mass rather than building it. Ideally, you should eat about 0.05 ounces of protein for each pound you weigh. Going over that too far can make the body create more glucose and keep your body out of ketosis.

How will I know I'm in ketosis and burning fat?

There are some lab tests and test strips that can be used to determine if you are in ketosis. You can pay to have your blood, urine or breath tested. But your body will give you certain signals that it's in the state of ketosis and the body is burning fat. Here are some of the ways your body will tell you it's resetting:

- Thirst Increases – You may start to experience more thirst or have a dry mouth. You can remedy this by making sure you are hydrated well.
- Urination Increases – Acetoacetate, one of the ketones, tends to build up in the urine. This is one reason there is a urine test that can be used to determine if you are in ketosis. But, the buildup of acetoacetate will also increase your need to urinate.
- Funny Smelling Breath – Acetone is another ketone. This ketone will escape the body through the breath. The result of this is an odd smell to your breath. It may smell kind of fruity, or it may smell more like nail polish remover. This same odor may come out in your sweat as well.
- Reduced Appetite – Many times people in ketosis experience greatly reduced hunger. This can occur because of the body being able to use up fat that has been stored. Once the Keto reset occurs, many only feel they need to eat a meal or two a day.
- More Energy – At first, it's possible you may feel tired because your body is making a huge adjustment. Later, you should feel a huge shift in energy levels. Some people who are in ketosis may even experience a feeling of euphoria.

How long will it take for the body to reach ketosis?

Each person is different and has a unique metabolism. This makes it difficult to put a single measure on how long it will take for your body to start burning fat, or be in ketosis. There are several things that may go into the mix. For instance, it may depend on your body's insulin resistance, or how active you are. Other factors that influence how quickly your body adjusts into the state of ketosis may be your body type and the specific foods you are eating. For some people, ketosis begins in as little as two days. For others though, it might be as long as ten days before the body fully adjusts. Generally, ketosis will not happen if you eat more than 30 grams of carbs each day. However, each person is different. Generally, the quickest way to get to a state of ketosis is to consume less than 20 grams of carbohydrates a day.

Is there really a "Keto flu"?

Some people may experience what is called, "Keto flu" when they first start the eating plan. Ketosis can have a diuretic effect and cause you to urinate more. If you are not hydrated properly you may experience headaches or brain fog. It's important to make sure you are replacing the electrolytes the body gets rid of through the urine. First of all, stay hydrated. Secondly eat foods with salt to help you with the transition into ketosis. Bacon, salted nuts and deli meat are all low carb, salty foods to help keep your system balanced out during the process.

It is also possible to experience some changes with your bowels because of the dietary changes. Drinking more water can be helpful. But you may also want to consume more coconut oil, choose vegetables with fiber or take a magnesium supplement to help. This is a natural process when you make changes to your diet.

Allowable Foods & Non-Allowable Foods

To achieve maximum results, it all comes down to what you eat. You may be wondering how this works and what foods you should or should not eat in order to reboot your metabolism and achieve a Keto reset. There are definitely some foods that need to be avoided, but there are also lots of foods allowed. Where in the world do you start, right? First, let's start with the food groups you need to focus on, and then we will break down each group into specific information about what to eat or avoid. Here are the basic food groups:

- *Fats/Oils*: The goal with eating fats is to get most of them from natural sources such as nuts or meat. Then you can supplement with other fats like butter, coconut oil and olive oil.
- *Proteins*: Consuming too much protein on a Ketogenic plan can have a negative effect, but you do need some. Try to eat meats that are natural with no sugar added. The best choices are grass fed, pasture raised and organic.
- *Vegetables*: Best choices for vegetable consumption are leafy green veggies. It won't matter if they are fresh or frozen.
- *Dairy Foods*: Most dairy items are good. Just be sure to buy items that are full-fat. Harder cheeses usually have less carbs, making them a better choice when it comes to cheese purchases.
- *Seeds & Nuts*: Use seeds and nuts in moderation. They will provide texture to the diet. When choosing nuts, go with those fattier options like almonds and macadamia nuts.
- *Drinks*: Keep it simple, and drink mostly water. Stevia flavorings are good or add lemon or lime juice if you want additional flavorings.

Now let's break down each of these groups and talk about specific foods so you can develop your own eating plan. We'll take an in depth look at each category and discuss the best food choices and the forbidden ones as well.

Fats/Oils

The cornerstone of the Keto diet is comprised of healthy fats. You want to keep your body in a state of ketosis, and to do that, you'll have to supply it with plenty of fats to break down for fuel. You want to give it plenty of fats for fuel, so it will use them instead of using protein or carbs. In fact, about 70% of your total caloric intake needs to be fat. However, it's important to note that you want high quality fats, this means that the source of fats matters. This is actually one of the best things about the keto diet, fats are filling and taste good! Just make sure you get the right fats. There are different types of fats including saturated, monounsaturated, and polyunsaturated. But how do you know which ones to choose? Here is a simple guide:

- **Saturated and Monounsaturated Fats:** Eat these types of fats.
- **Polyunsaturated Fats:** Natural polyunsaturated fats like what you find in fish and animal proteins are good for you, eat them! However, if polyunsaturated fats are processed like in margarine spreads are not "heart healthy." Avoid these types of processed fats.

Monounsaturated and Saturated Fats

Here are some good fats you should consume:
- Natural butters Including butter, ghee, cocoa butter or coconut butter
- Egg Yolks (It's worth the extra expense to purchase pasture-raised eggs)
- Oils including coconut oil, MCT oil, avocado oil and olive oil
- Nuts, seeds, and nut butters (choose nuts with higher fat content like almonds or macadamia nuts)
- Fatty Fish
- Avocados

Red meat, lard, coconut oil, palm oil, eggs, ghee and eggs contain saturated fats. Remember to choose organic foods when possible. Use saturated fats like coconut oil or butter for cooking. The bulk of your fat intake should be from monounsaturated and saturated fats. Medium-chain triglycerides or MCTs, are saturated fats that are digested easily by the body. When the body ingests MCTs, they pass directly to the liver and are used for an immediate energy source. Coconut oil contains the largest amount of MCTs, but they are also found in smaller amounts in palm oil and butter. Athletes often use MCTs to help improve their performance. If your stomach can tolerate pure MCT oil, then you may want to purchase the supplement. Monounsaturated fatty acid or MUFA is found in olives, beef, nuts and avocados. They are known to help prevent heart disease. Oils that are high in MUFA are best used cold. Extra virgin olive oil, macadamia nut oil and avocado oil can all be used cold.

Polyunsaturated Fats

Remember that you want to maintain a good balance of omega 3s and omega 6s. These are both essential fatty acids you need in your diet. There are several reasons they are so important including brain and nerve function. They are also great for reducing a variety of diseases like heart disease, type 2 diabetes, and Alzheimer's. Omega-6 is beneficial and even necessary, but consuming too much can cause inflammation. Just be cautious when consuming some of the foods containing higher amounts of Omega-6 such as plant oils like sunflower or corn oil; or peanuts. Try to focus on consuming omega 3s in different types of fish like tuna, trout, mackerel or salmon. You may also want to take a fish oil supplement; just be sure it is of high quality. Remember that some nuts can have more carbs especially pistachios, cashews and almonds.

Proteins

Maintaining Keto means eating proteins only in moderation. Continue to monitor protein content when consuming meats and other protein sources like eggs. If you consume too much protein, the body may switch to breaking down proteins for fuel rather than fats. This can stop ketosis altogether, or at least decrease it. If you choose to eat meat that is leaner, try to include a side dish or sauce that contains fat along with it. When selecting meat, go with options that are grass-fed or pasture-raised. Also be careful about eating meats that have ingredients that have undergone processing. Cured meats for instance, have additional sugars. Eating processed meats increases your sugar and carb intake. Here are some guidelines for consuming proteins:

- Beef cuts should be fattier and might include steak, roast, beef, or veal
- Poultry – think about darker portions as they are fattier. You can try chicken, duck, turkey, quail or other wild game.
- Pork options may include bacon, pork loin, tenderloin, ham, chops, or ground pork. Again, avoid processed forms of pork like sausage.
- Fish choices might include tuna, trout, mackerel, salmon, cod, halibut, mahi-mahi or catfish.
- Shellfish includes lobster, mussels, crab, clams and oysters.
- Organ meats can provide protein, including liver, kidney, offal, tongue and heart.
- Eggs prepared any way including boiled, deviled, scrambled and fried. Remember to use whole eggs.

- Lamb
- Goat
- Nut butters are a natural form of protein, and need to be unsweetened. Try to stick to macadamia or almond nut butters. Peanuts are legumes that are high in omega 3s so consume them sparingly.

Fruits and Veggies

Vegetables are an essential part of a healthy, balanced Keto diet, but not just any vegetables. First, you'll want to eliminate veggies that are high in sugar. This group of vegetables are not balanced nutritionally. You may have already guessed that you want to go with vegetables that are leafy and dark. This of course, includes vegetables like spinach and kale. Ideally, vegetables that are grown above the grown are cruciferous, green and leafy are the best choices. When it is possible, you'll also want to choose organically grown vegetables and fruits to avoid pesticide residue. Nutritionally, vegetables grown organically or non-organically are the same. You can also choose from either fresh or frozen vegetables.

As for veggies that grow below the ground, they can be consumed, but use moderation. Watch how many carbs they have. Underground vegetables like onions are good to use for adding flavor, like onions for example. But typically, you only need a half of an onion for a whole pot of soup. When choosing vegetables, carefully monitor carbohydrates and portion them by carb content.

In general, veggies are good, but watch their carb counts. Eating just a single serving of a starchy vegetable like a potato can put you over the limit of carbs for the day. These vegetables and fruits should be limited because they have more carbs:

- Nightshades like tomato, peppers and eggplants
- Root veggies including onions, garlic, mushrooms, squash and parsnips
- Berries including blackberries, blueberries and raspberries
- Citrus fruit including limes, lemon, orange juice
- Starchy vegetables and large fruit should be totally avoided including bananas and potatoes

There are many vegetables with low carbs you can choose. Remember your best options are green and leafy. Choose options like broccoli, cauliflower and kale. You can also make noodle substitutes from zucchini to reduce your carbs. Spaghetti squash is a natural, low-carb substitute for spaghetti. Other low-carb nutritious options include:

- Romaine Lettuce
- Bok Choy
- Brussels Sprouts
- Swiss Chard
- Kale
- Spinach
- Cucumber
- Cauliflower
- Green Beans

What about fruit consumption?

Fruits can be eaten, but they need to be very limited and in small amounts due to their high sugar content. If you eat fruit, organic is the best choice, but not essential. You may choose from either fresh or frozen, just be sure it's all-natural fruit without other ingredients. Some low-sugar fruit options include:

- Mulberries
- Cherries
- Blueberries
- Strawberries
- Raspberries
- Cranberries

Dairy Products

Dairy products can be consumed on Keto. For many people, dairy helps balance out meals. Just be sure to watch two things the number of carbs and the amount of protein. Since you need fat to achieve ketosis, you will want to choose cheeses that are full fat instead of low-fat or fat free options. Keeping an eye on the number of carbs cheese servings contain, you may want to include these dairy products with some of your meals.

- Heavy cream
- Greek yogurt
- Mayonnaise (homemade if possible)
- Cheese spreads like crème fraiche, sour cream, cream cheese and cottage cheese
- Soft cheeses like mozzarella, Monterey jack, blue, or Colby
- Hard cheeses like parmesan, Swiss, feta and aged cheddar

Dairy sources provide extra fats and can be used in dips and to create other fatty sides. Be sure to read the ingredients because many products have added sugar.

Sauces and Condiments

You will want to be careful to check the labels on condiments and sauces. Many of them contain added sugars. If you want Keto to be most effective, you'll want to be stricter on what you allow and disallow. For the most part, you will want to avoid pre-made condiments and sauces because they may contain added sweeteners or sugars that could sabotage your efforts. You may want to make your own gravies and sauces, but if you do make sure to use xanthan gum or guar for a thickening agent. There is also a lot on the market today that are higher in fat and lower in carbs. If you make sauces, consider browning butter, beurre blanc of hollandaise. It's also worth noting that condiments and sauces can vary greatly between brands so be sure to read the labels. In general, you could consider using these condiments:

- Ketchup (low or no-sugar added version)
- Sauerkraut (no or low sugar added)
- Mustard
- Horseradish
- Relish (low sugar or no sugar)
- Worcestershire sauce
- Some Salad Dressings
- Some Flavored Syrups

Be sure to err on the side of caution when choosing pre-made condiments to use for Keto dieting. It's best to make your own gravies, sauces and condiments when you can. Always check and double check ingredient lists to be sure they comply with Keto standards.

Ketogenic Diet Recipes

If you are just starting on your Keto journey, it can be difficult to make the switch to a low carb, low protein, high fat diet. You may even be thinking you will have to give up your favorite dishes and snacks. You'll be glad to hear that in most cases, you can make a few ingredient changes and make your favorites Keto-friendly. The good news is, you are bound to find some new favorites while maintaining ketosis. Here are lots of Ketogenic recipes broken into several categories including breakfast, meat, poultry, seafood, appetizers, main courses and snacks. Take these great ideas to your Keto kitchen! Whether you are just getting started or have been eating a Ketogenic diet for some time, you will find these delicious keto recipes useful, easy and tasty. Enjoy!

Breakfast

Cauliflower Hash Browns with Onions and Chives

Cook Time: 25 minutes
Servings: 2

Ingredients:
- 2 cups of "riced" cauliflower (approximately half of a large head of cauliflower)
- 1 large egg
- Salt and pepper, to taste
- 1 tbsp diced onion
- 1 tsp diced green pepper
- 1 tsp diced red pepper
- ½ tbsp olive oil
- Small block of onion and chive Cotswold cheese

Method:
1. Combine the cauliflower, egg, salt, pepper, onion, green and red peppers in a bowl. Stir until it is combined well.
2. Heat olive oil in a small pan over medium-high heat.
3. After the olive oil is hot, spoon half of the cauliflower mix into the oil. Using the spoon, flatten it out to about 1/3 inch thick. Smooth the edges.
4. Let it brown for about 4 to 5 minutes, just until it's crispy. Then flip it using a spatula.
5. While it is cooking, grate a very generous amount of the Cotswold cheese on top. Continue to let the hash browns cook until the cheese has melted. It should take 3 to 4 minutes.
6. Remove from the pan and repeat the steps with the other half of the batter.

Breakfast Bagels

Cook Time: About 20 minutes
Servings: 3

Ingredients:
- ¾ cup of almond flour
- 1 tsp xanthan gum
- 1 egg (large)
- 2 tbsp cream cheese
- 1 ½ cups grated mozzarella cheese
- 1 tbsp melted butter
- 1 tbsp sesame seeds

Optional (fillings):
- Pesto, cream cheese, arugula leaves and bacon

Method:
1. Preheat the oven to 390 degrees (F) and mix the almond flour and xanthan gum together in a bowl.
2. Add in the egg and mix it together until it is mixed well and forms a doughy ball.
3. Melt cream cheese and mozzarella cheese together over medium-low heat or in the microwave. Remove the cheese from the heat as soon as it is melted.
4. Add the melted mixed cheese into the almond flour mixture and knead well until it is completely mixed and well combined. The mozzarella will try to stick together in a ball, but keep kneading it until it is all thoroughly combined. Be sure that the xanthan gum is mixed throughout the dough. If the dough becomes stiff and hard to work with, microwave it for 10 to 20 seconds and continue mixing until it looks like a solid dough ball.
5. Split the ball of dough into three pieces and roll them out into round logs. If you do not have a donut pan, make each log into a round circle and place them on a baking tray. You may choose to make the dough into three balls, then roll them out and use a small cookie cutter to remove the centers so they are shaped like a bagel.
6. Melt the butter and brush it over the top of the bagels. Sprinkle on sesame seeds to your liking or use a topping of your choice. The butter will help ensure the seeds stick to the bagel. Garlic powder or onion powder make a savory addition as well.
7. Bake the bagels for approximately 18 minutes. The top should be golden brown. Once they are done, remove from the oven and allow them to cool.

8. If you like toasted bagels, cut them in half and put them back in the oven until they are toasted.
9. Top the toasted bagel with your favorite topping. My favorite is to spread cream cheese, cover that in pesto, add some arugula leaves and a couple of slices of smoke salmon. Net carbs are just under 6g.

Baked Bacon Omelet

Cook Time: Less than 30 minutes
Servings: 1

Ingredients:
- 5 1/3 oz. bacon, cut into small pieces
- 2 oz. fresh spinach
- 3 oz. butter
- 2 medium or large eggs
- Salt and/or pepper, to taste
- 1 tbsp fresh chives, finely chopped (optional)

Method:
1. Preheat oven to 400 degrees (F) and grease a single serving sized baking dish.
2. Fry the bacon and spinach in the butter.
3. Whisk eggs until they become frothy. Then stir in the bacon and spinach mixture. Include any of the fat left in the skillet.
4. Add salt, pepper and fresh chopped chives to personal preference and taste.
5. Pour egg mixture into the baking dish and back until the top is golden brown (about 20 minutes).
6. Remove from the oven and let it cool for several minutes before serving.

Poached Eggs in Spiced Tomato Sauce

Cook Time: About 45 Minutes
Servings: 2

Ingredients:
- 1 tbsp grass-fed organic ghee
- 1 white onion, chopped
- 3 cloves of garlic, minced
- 1 serrano pepper, chopped
- 1 red bell pepper, chopped
- 1 tsp cumin
- 1 tsp paprika
- ¼ tsp chili powder
- 3 tomatoes (medium sized), chopped
- 5 to 6 eggs
- ¼ tsp salt, to taste
- ¼ tsp pepper, to taste
- Fresh cilantro for garnish (optional)

Method:
1. Heat ghee over a medium heat and add onions. Stir occasionally until they begin to turn golden brown. (10-15 minutes).
2. After the onions are softened, add garlic and the Serrano pepper. Let it cook for a few minutes.
3. Then add the red bell pepper and lower the heat. Stir occasionally and cook for about 10 minutes.
4. Add other spices and stir. Then add the chopped tomatoes. Bring to a simmer and cook until the tomato starts to thicken into a sauce consistency.
5. Carefully crack eggs into the tomato sauce and season with salt and pepper. Cover and cook for about 5 minutes, or until the eggs are done. Cooking longer will yield "harder' yolks. Reduce cooking time for softer poached eggs.
6. Sprinkle with fresh cilantro and serve.

Brussels Sprouts and Eggs Hash

Cook Time: Under 30 minutes
Servings: 3

Ingredients:

- Brussels sprouts (about 12 ounces)
- 2 oz. bacon
- 2 garlic cloves, minced
- 2 shallots, minced
- 1 ½ tbsp apple cider vinegar
- 1 tbsp butter
- 3 eggs
- Kosher salt and cracked black pepper

Method:

1. Slice Brussels sprouts into thin slices then set aside.
2. Cook bacon in a skillet until it is crisp then remove from pan.
3. Add garlic and shallots to the bacon grease and cook for about 30 seconds then add the Brussels sprouts.
4. Stir in the apple cider vinegar and sauté for about 5 minutes or until the Brussels sprouts are tender.
5. Put the bacon back in the pan and stir. Cook for about 3 to 5 minutes until the edges of the sprouts start to brown.
6. Create a "well" in the middle of the pan by moving the mix to the edges.
7. Add butter, then crack eggs into the center and continue to cook until eggs are cooked to the desired degree.
8. Remove from heat. Serve and enjoy!

Shrimp Omelet

Cook Time: 10 minutes
Servings: 2

Ingredients:
- ¼ onion
- 4 grape tomatoes
- 1 tbsp olive oil or coconut oil
- Pinch of salt
- Handful of fresh spinach
- 10 medium to large shrimp
- ¼ tsp cayenne pepper (optional)
- 1 tbsp Sriracha (optional)
- 6 eggs
- 1 sprig of parsley

Method:
1. Chop up the onion and cut the tomatoes into halves.
2. Place a pan over a medium heat to heat the oil, then add onions and sprinkle salt. Place the tomatoes face down to toast them slightly.
3. Once the onions are translucent, toss in the spinach and allow it to wilt. This allows room for the shrimp.
4. Add in the shrimp, spices (optional) and once the spinach is wilted down.
5. Add the eggs; mix and pour them over the spinach mixture or make a sunny side-up. Put a lid on the pan so the omelet will cook on top too.
6. Cook eggs long enough for the consistency you prefer. The longer you cook it, the less runny the eggs will be.
7. Once the omelet is done, add parsley as garnish.

Hash Browns / Spaghetti Squash

Cook Time: about 15 minutes (using cooked spaghetti squash)
Serves: 1

Ingredients:
- 1 cup cooked spaghetti squash threads
- 1 tbsp butter, coconut oil or ghee
- Sea salt

Method:
1. Place the cooked spaghetti squash threads in a towel and wring out excess moisture. You will notice the squash shrinks in size.
2. Heat oil over a medium/high heat in a skillet.
3. Add drained spaghetti squash and press down with a spatula until it creates a thin, even layer on the bottom of the skillet. Sprinkle the top with salt to taste.
4. Cook until first side is browned then gently flip.
5. Cook on the other side until brown, sprinkle with salt to taste and serve.

Turkey Breakfast Wrap

Cook Time: About 25 minutes
Serving: 2

Ingredients:
- 2 slices bacon
- 2 tbsp coconut oil for cooking
- 2 eggs
- 2 large leaves of romaine lettuce – or 2 avocado slices
- 2 turkey breast slices, cooked

Method:
1. Cook the sliced bacon to your desired level of crispiness.
2. Scramble the eggs in coconut oil.
3. Make the two breakfast wraps by putting half the bacon, scrambled eggs and lettuce on each slice of turkey. Fold and eat. Yummy!

Sausage Breakfast Sandwich

Cook Time: 20 minutes
Serving: 1

Ingredients:

- 2 sausage patties (cook your own or precooked)
- 1 tbsp cream cheese
- 2 tbsp sharp cheddar cheese
- ¼ tsp Sriracha powder
- 1 medium egg
- ¼ avocado, sliced
- Salt and pepper, to taste

Method:

1. Cook sausage patties in a skillet over medium heat (Or according to package instructions).
2. Melt cream cheese and sharp cheddar cheese together. Microwave for 20 to 30 seconds or use a double broiler.
3. Mix Sriracha powder with melted cheese and set aside.
4. Scramble the egg and make a small omelet.
5. Fill the egg omelet with cheese mixture.
6. Add omelet and avocado slices between sausage patties to form a breakfast sandwich.

Cauliflower Hash Brown Waffles

Cook Time: 15 to 20 minutes
Serves: 2

Ingredients:
- 1 head of cauliflower
- 2 eggs
- 1 bunch of scallions, diced
- 8 oz. of cubed ham
- 2 tbsp olive oil
- 2 to 3 tbsp sharp cheddar (optional)
- ½ tsp salt and pepper, to taste
- Fresh cilantro, parsley or basil (garnish)

Method:
1. Separate florets and stems from the rest of the cauliflower and leaves. Using a food processor or grater, create a pile of small cauliflower shavings.
2. Place cauliflower in a bowl and add all the other ingredients (except garnish) and stir it together until mixed.
3. Pour ½ of the mixture onto a well-greased, pre-heated waffle iron. Cook on medium-high heat until golden brown. Carefully remove from waffle iron using a spatula and a fork.
4. Repeat with the other half of the mixture.
5. Add garnish and enjoy!

No-Crust Spinach Quiche

Cook Time: 40 minutes
Servings: 4

Ingredients:
- 1 tbsp coconut oil
- 1 onion, chopped
- 1 package frozen spinach, (chopped) thawed and drained
- 8 eggs
- 3 cups shredded cheese
- ¼ tsp sea salt
- 1/8 tsp black pepper

Method:
1. Preheat the oven to 350 degrees (F). Grease a 9-inch pie pan with coconut oil.
2. Heat onions in the coconut oil over medium heat. Cook until onions are soft, then stir in the spinach and cook until all the moisture is gone.
3. Combine eggs, cheese and salt/pepper in a bowl. Blend in the spinach mixture.
4. Pour into baking pan. Bake for 30 minutes.

Salmon Breakfast Balls

Cook Time: 30 minutes
Serves: 2

Ingredients:

- 2 eggs
- 4 oz. sliced smoked salmon
- ½ tbsp salted butter
- 2 tbsp fresh chives, chopped
- Salt and pepper, to taste

For Hollandaise sauce:

- 2 tbsp salted butter
- 1 egg yolk (without the white)
- 2 tsp freshly squeezed lemon juice
- ¼ tsp Dijon mustard
- Salt, to taste
- ½ tbsp water (a little more if needed)

Method:

1. Set ingredients needed for the hollandaise sauce out so they can reach room temperature.
2. Boil the two eggs for salmon balls. They need to be hard boiled since the hollandaise will be added to them.
3. Dice the salmon slices up and preheat a pan over high heat.
4. Add two teaspoons butter to the pan.
5. Once the butter is melted and hot, put about half of the salmon in it and fry until they are crispy and crunchy. Then set them aside.
6. Peel the boiled eggs and mash them up with a fork.

For hollandaise sauce:

7. Put a cup or two of water on the stove and allow it to simmer.
8. Melt the 2 tablespoons of butter for 30 to 60 seconds in the microwave. It should be melted, but not hot. Set butter aside.
9. In a large bowl, whisk the egg yolk, lemon juice, mustard and a pinch of the salt. Mix it until you see some bubbles.
10. Put the bowl over the simmering pot so you have a double broiler. Don't let the water touch the bottom of the bowl.
11. Whisk the mixture continuously until it begins to get thick.

12. Remove the bowl from the pot, and slowly pour in the melted butter and continue to stir with the whisk. Continue stirring to avoid the mixture clumping.
13. After the butter is added, put the bowl back on the pot and let it thicken a bit more.
14. Once the sauce is thick, remove it and set it aside and allow it to cool off to room temperature. If it's too thick, add a little bit of water.
15. Then mix the raw salmon, half the chives, and the hollandaise and mix it all with the mashed up egg. It should become very firm. Adjust the hollandaise so that it does not too wet.
16. Once it is all mixed up – make it into four similarly sized balls. Mix crispy salmon and chives together and roll the four balls in it to coat them.
17. Serve and enjoy!

Breakfast Salad

Cook Time: 25 minutes
Serves: 1

Ingredients:
- 2 eggs
- 2 to 4 pieces of bacon
- 1 ripe avocado
- 1 medium tomato
- Lemon juice
- Salt and pepper, to taste

Method:
1. Boil the two eggs and fry the bacon.
2. Chop up the avocado and the tomato.
3. Chop up the fried bacon. Peel the boiled eggs and chop.
4. Mix all the ingredients together with lemon juice and add salt and pepper to taste.

Chorizo Sausage, Goat Cheese, Spinach Omelet

Cook Time: 40 minutes
Servings: 2

Ingredients:

- 4 oz. of chorizo sausage
- 4 eggs
- 1 tbsp water
- ½ tbsp butter
- 2 cups baby spinach
- 2 oz. fresh goat cheese crumbles
- ¼ salsa Verde (optional)
- Avocado slices

Method:

1. Remove the chorizo sausage from its casing and fry it in a skillet until it is fully cooked.
2. Beat the eggs and water in a small bowl.
3. Remove the chorizo from the skillet using a slotted spoon. Sit the sausage aside.
4. Using the same pan, melt the butter over a low heat. Add the eggs to the pan.
5. While the eggs cook, place the sausage, spinach and goat cheese on half the side of the eggs. Cook for 3 minutes on low heat. The eggs should be slightly firm.
6. Fold the empty side of the eggs over on top of the loaded side.
7. Cover the pan and let it cook on low heat just until the eggs are cooked all the way through. If they seem to be cooking too quickly, turn the heat off and cover the pan, and let it set for about 10 minutes.
8. Serve with salsa Verde or avocado slices, or both!

Meat

Salisbury Steak

Cook Time: approximately 35 minutes
Servings: About 4

Ingredients:
- 1 ½ lb. of ground beef
- 1 medium egg
- 1 finely chopped large shallot
- 2 tsp Worcestershire sauce
- 1 ¼ tsp kosher salt
- 5 tbsp unsalted butter
- 8-12 oz. mushrooms (crimini or button)
- ½ cup red wine
- 1 ½ cups beef stock

Method:
1. Preheat oven to 350 degrees (F).
2. Mix together the beef, egg, shallot, Worcestershire sauce and salt in a large mixing bowl. Once it is mixed thoroughly, shape into four round or oval patties.
3. Melt 2 tablespoons of butter in a skillet over medium/high heat. As soon as the butter melts but before it browns, add the beef patties. Brown them for 3 to 4 minutes on each side.
4. Once they are browned, place them in a baking dish and cover with foil. Bake in oven for about 10 minutes or until they are fully cooked.
5. Add another tablespoon of butter to the same skillet along with the mushrooms. Cook mushrooms until they are soft and brown, stir them as little as possible. Season to taste with salt and pepper, then remove from skillet and set aside.
6. Add red wine to the same skillet and simmer over a medium/high heat until it is reduced by half. This usually takes only 3 to 5 minutes. Add beef broth and simmer for about 12 minutes or until it is reduced by half. Turn heat to low and whisk in 2 tablespoons of butter. Allow it to simmer until the sauce has the desired consistency.
7. Remove meat patties from oven and cover with mushrooms. Drizzle the sauce over the top. Serve with your favorite side.

Zucchini Beef Stir Fry

Cook Time: About 15 minutes
Serves: 1

Ingredients:
- Cut of beef that can be chopped into strips (thin steak)
- 1 medium zucchini
- 2 tbsp avocado oil (or coconut oil or olive oil)
- ¼ cup gluten free tamari soy sauce
- Pinch of cilantro
- 1 clove of garlic

Method:
1. Chop beef into strips. Slice against the grain to make the meat easier to eat.
2. Peel zucchini and chop it into strips that are about the same size as the beef strips.
3. Pour your choice of oil into a skillet and turn to high heat, then add the beef strips. Sauté until the beef is browned.
4. After the beef is browned, add zucchini strips and sauté until they start to soften. Then add soy sauce, cilantro and garlic.
5. Continue to sauté for about 2 more minutes and serve while warm.

Keto Cabbage Casserole

Cook Time: Less than 45 minutes
Servings: 4

Ingredients:
- 1.5 lb. green cabbage
- 5 1/3 oz. butter
- 1 tsp salt
- 1 tsp onion powder
- ¼ tsp black pepper
- 2 tbsp Tex-Mex or Taco seasoning
- 1 tbsp white wine vinegar
- 1 lb. ground beef
- Salt and pepper, to taste
- 2/3 lb. shredded cheddar cheese
- 5-6 oz. lettuce or leafy greens

Method:
1. Preheat oven to 400 degrees (F) while you shred the cabbage with a processor or finely chop it with a knife.
2. Use 3 ounces of the butter to fry the chopped cabbage in a wok or skillet until it's soft, but not turning brown. This may take about 10 minutes.
3. Add all the spices and wine vinegar. Continue to fry and stir for a couple minutes, then set it aside on a plate.
4. Melt the rest of the butter in the same skillet or wok. Sauté the beef on medium high setting until the juices are almost gone, then lower to medium low heat.
5. Add the cooked cabbage back in and sauté for a couple minutes. Remove from heat and add salt and pepper if desired.
6. Stir about 2/3 of the cheese into the cabbage mix and place it all in a baking dish. Then sprinkle the rest of the cheese on top and bake for 15 to 20 minutes or until the cheese is lightly browned.
7. Serve over the fresh greens.

Crispy Pork Bites

Cook Time: 45 minutes
Servings: 3

Ingredients:
- 10 ½ oz. thin pork belly strips (or about 300g of other pork)
- Salt
- 1 tbsp butter
- ¼ onion, diced
- 4 tbsp heavy cream
- 1.75 oz. blue cheese

Method:
1. Preheat oven to 475 degrees (F), or its highest bake setting.
2. Place pork belly strips in an oven dish and rub with salt until they are covered thinly with salt.
3. Bake pork strips for about 35 minutes. Watch them closely until they are crispy brown colored and the fat has rendered out.
4. In another pan, caramelize the onions in butter, but heat them slowly on medium heat so they will be sweet.
5. After the onions are cooked, add cream (without reducing the heat).
6. As soon as the cream is warm, add the blue cheese and wait for it to melt. Then turn the heat up to high for about a minute. Then pour the mixture into a dish.
7. Remove pork from the oven (if you haven't already) and let it cool down on a paper towel, then cut it into bite-size chunks.
8. Put toothpicks in the pork pieces and dip them into the dip. Delicious!

Meat Stuffed Zucchini Boats

Cook Time: 45 minutes
Servings: 3

Ingredients:
- ½ onion
- ½ tbsp butter
- 0.7 lb. ground meat (beef or pork)
- 1 medium egg
- 3 to 4 zucchini depending on their size
- ½ cup grated Gouda cheese
- ¼ cup grated mimolette cheese (optional)
- 1/3 cup grated mozzarella cheese
- 2 tbsp Parmesan cheese

Method:
1. Cut up the onion and fry it in the butter for about two minutes.
2. Add the ground meat and fry for an additional three minutes. Make sure to break the meat into small pieces while it is frying.
3. Place the fried meat and onions in a bowl and add the egg, then mix them together well.
4. Cut the zucchini squash in half and clean out the seeds. Place the meat mixture in the zucchini "boats" and bake at 200 degrees (F) for 15 minutes.
5. Mix the cheeses together (gouda, mimolette and mozzarella) then sprinkle it on top of the boats and bake for an additional 5 minutes.
6. Sprinkle the Parmesan cheese on top and bake for one or two more minutes. Let cool – then enjoy!

Keto Beef Stroganoff

Cook Time: 45 minutes
Servings: 6

Ingredients:
- 1 tsp salt
- ½ tsp garlic powder
- 1.5 lb. cauliflower
- 1 lb. of ground beef
- ½ cup fresh chopped onion
- ½ cup sliced mushrooms (skip this and save some carbs!)
- ½ cup white wine
- ¼ cup cream
- 2 oz. shredded Monterey jack cheese
- 1 cup sour cream
- Salt and pepper, to taste
- Fresh parsley (garnish)

Method:
1. Bring to boil two cups of water, and put 1 tsp salt and garlic powder.
2. Add cut up cauliflower, reduce the heat and cover. Simmer until cauliflower is tender.
3. Drain cauliflower and set aside.
4. Cook the beef and onion in a skillet until the beef is thoroughly cooked. Then add mushrooms if using them.
5. Drain fat off beef and blot with a towel to remove grease.
6. Add the cauliflower, wine and cream to the beef mix.
7. Stir in the cheese and sour cream.
8. Heat until hot all the way through. Add salt and pepper to taste and sprinkle with parsley for a garnish.

Jalapeno Cheddar Beef or Turkey Burgers

Cook Time: 30-45 minutes based on cooking method
Servings: 4 burgers

Ingredients:
- 2 oz. shredded cheddar cheese
- 4 tbsp cream cheese
- ¼ tsp garlic powder
- 1 fresh seeded jalapeno pepper
- 28 oz. beef or turkey
- 2 tbsp minced onions
- Salt and pepper, to taste
- 1 tbsp olive oil

Method:
1. Preheat oven or grill to high setting.
2. Combine cheddar cheese, cream cheese, garlic powder and chopped or diced jalapeno in a small bowl.
3. Mix meat, minced onion and salt and pepper together in another bowl, then divide into four even pieces.
4. Put ¼ of the cheese mixture in the middle of each patty and wrap the meat around the cheese so it's totally covered. Repeat for the other 3 burgers.
5. Brush the outside of each burger with oil.
6. Grill the burgers for 6 to 7 minutes on each side over medium heat until cooked completely.
7. OR Broil burgers on a pan covered with foil. Place the pan about 6 inches from the broiler and broil for 5 to 6 minutes on each side. Cook completely.

Crock Pot Pulled Pork

Cook Time: 8 hours (with 10+ minutes prep time)
Serves: 4

Ingredients:
- 2 tbsp paprika
- 2 tbsp chili powder
- 2 tbsp cumin
- 1 tbsp white pepper
- 1 tbsp black pepper
- 2 tsp cayenne
- 2 tsp dry mustard
- 2 tsp sea salt
- 3 ½ lb. pork shoulder roast

Method:
1. Combine all the spices and mix thoroughly.
2. Rub the pork with the spice mixture. Make sure it is evenly coated and in every little crevice.
3. Wrap the rubbed pork tightly in plastic wrap and let it set in the fridge overnight.
4. Unwrap the pork after it has set and place it in your crock pot or slow cooker.
5. Cook on low for 8 hours.
6. Use in any recipe calling for pulled pork.

Eggplant N Beef Pizza

Cook Time: about an hour
Servings: 4

Ingredients:
- 2 eggplants
- 1/3 cup olive oil
- 2 cloves of garlic
- 1 yellow onion
- ¾ lb. ground beef
- 7 oz. tomato sauce
- 1 tsp salt
- ½ tsp pepper
- ½ tsp cinnamon (optional)
- 2/3 lb. grated cheese
- 4 tbsp fresh oregano, chopped

Method:
1. Preheat oven to 400 degrees (F).
2. Slice the eggplants long-wise so the slices are about 1/3 to ½ inch in thickness.
3. Coat both sides with olive oil and bake for about 20 minutes, or until they are barely browned.
4. Sauté' garlic and onion in olive oil until soft, this should take 3 or 4 minutes.
5. Add beef and cook until thoroughly done. Then add tomato sauce and salt and pepper. Let meat mixture simmer for about 10 minutes, or until it is good and warm.
6. Spread the meat mixture over the toasted eggplant slices. Sprinkle cheese and oregano on top. Place back into the oven for about 10 minutes, or until the cheese is melted.
7. Serve with a leafy, green salad and enjoy!

Bacon-Cheeseburger Casserole

Cook Time: 45 minutes
Servings: 12

Ingredients:
- 2 lb. ground beef
- 2 large garlic cloves
- ½ tsp onion powder
- 1 lb. bacon (cooked and chopped)
- 8 eggs
- 1 6-oz. can tomato paste
- 1 cup heavy cream
- ½ tsp salt
- ¼ tsp pepper
- 12 oz. cheddar cheese (grated)

Method:
1. Cook and brown the beef, garlic and onion powder. Drain grease and stir in bacon pieces.
2. Spread the meat mixture on the bottom of a 9x13 casserole pan.
3. Whisk together eggs, tomato paste, cream, salt and pepper in a medium sized bowl.
4. Stir 8 ounces of cheddar cheese into the egg mixture then pour it over the meat mixture in the casserole dish. Top with the other 4 ounces of cheese.
5. Bake in a 350-degree (F) oven for 30 to 35 minutes or until the top is a pretty golden brown.

Note: You can reduce the number of eggs and increase the amount of beef.

Beef 'N "Rice"

Cook Time: 35 minutes
Servings: 6

Ingredients:
- 4 cups of cauliflower ("riced" in food processor)
- 1 tbsp butter or coconut oil
- 1 small onion, chopped
- 2 cups of mushrooms (optional to save carbs)
- 1 garlic clove, minced
- 1 lb. grass-fed ground beef
- Salt and pepper, to taste
- 16 oz. of salsa or tomato sauce (salsa is lower in carbs)
- 4 oz. cheddar cheese

Method:
1. Use the processor to grind cauliflower into a "rice" consistency.
2. Melt the butter in a large pan and then add onions and mushrooms if you want mushrooms. Sauté until the onions are tender. This should take about 5 minutes.
3. Add the garlic and continue to sauté until it's fragrant, about a minute.
4. Add the cauliflower rice and stir until it is coated with the butter. Simmer until cauliflower is cooked, around 5 minutes. Remove from pan and set it aside.
5. Cook the beef using the same pan until it is done and no pink shows, then drain off the extra fat.
6. Add the cauliflower mixture to the meat, and season with salt and pepper.
7. Pour in the tomato sauce. Top with the grated cheese (or guacamole). Let it stand long enough to melt the cheese.

Beef and Zucchini Burgers

Cook Time: 25 minutes
Servings: 6

Ingredients:
- 1 ½ lb. of ground beef
- 1 ½ cups of grated zucchini
- ½ tsp salt
- ½ tsp pepper
- 2 tsp cumin
- ½ tsp cinnamon
- ½ cup sour cream
- 5 oz. feta cheese
- 2 tbsp lemon juice
- 12 lettuce leaves
- Hot sauce (optional)

Method:
1. Mix the beef, zucchini, salt, pepper, cumin and cinnamon together in a bowl.
2. Shape the meat mixture into 12 small patties.
3. Preheat over to 450 degrees (F), or heat up the outdoor grill.
4. Brown both sides of the burgers in a skillet, then transfer to the oven and cook 8 minutes on each side.
5. In a small bowl, whisk the sour cream and about 4 ounces of the feta cheese. Stir in the lemon juice and then set it aside.
6. Place the cooked burgers on lettuce leaves and top each one with 3 tablespoons of the feta cheese sauce.
7. Crumble the remaining ounce or two of feta cheese over the top. Add hot sauce if preferred.

Poultry

Lettuce Wraps with Chicken Salad

Cook Time: 10 minutes
Servings: 4 to 6

Ingredients:
- 3 tbsp red hot sauce
- 3 tbsp mayonnaise
- 3 tbsp ranch dressing
- ¼ tsp garlic powder
- 2 ¼ cups cooked and cubed chicken
- ¼ cup diced red onion
- ½ cup diced celery
- 3 green onions, chopped
- ½ cup shredded or diced carrots
- Large leaf lettuce (Butter lettuce or green leaf lettuce or mixed greens)

Method:
1. Mix hot sauce, mayo, ranch dressing, and garlic powder together in a medium sized bowl.
2. Add chopped chicken, red onion and celery then mix until it's combined.
3. Serve chicken salad wrapped in lettuce or on a bed of greens. Top with green onions and carrots (Add more hot sauce for more flavor.)

Chicken Casserole

Cook Time: Less than an hour
Serves: 2-4

Ingredients:
- 1 cup of heavy cream
- 2 tbsp green pesto
- ½ lemon for juice
- 2 lb. of chicken thighs
- Salt and pepper, to taste
- 3 tbsp butter
- 4 oz. of cherry tomatoes
- 1 leek
- ¾ lb. cauliflower florets
- 7 oz. shredded cheese

Method:
1. Preheat oven to 400 degrees (F).
2. Mix cream with pesto and lemon juice.
3. Sprinkle salt and pepper on chicken thighs, then fry in the butter until the sides are golden brown.
4. Place chicken thighs in a baking dish, then pour the cream mixture over the thighs.
5. Chop the cherry tomatoes and leek then place on top of the chicken along with the cauliflower florets.
6. Sprinkle shredded cheese on the top and bake for about 30 minutes or until the chicken is cooked through.

Keto Chicken Pad Thai

Cook Time: About 30 minutes
Serves: 2-4

Ingredients:
- 1/8 tsp ginger
- 1/8 tsp garlic powder
- 1/8 tsp sea salt
- 1/8 tsp black pepper
- 2 lb. free-range chicken tender
- 2 tbsp peanut oil
- 3 large eggs
- 1/3 cup chicken broth
- 3 tbsp peanut butter
- 2 tbsp tamari
- ½ cup scallion, chopped
- 1 tsp red pepper flakes
- 2 cloves garlic, minced
- 1 tbsp rice vinegar
- 4 spiralized zucchini
- ½ cup bean sprouts
- 1 lime (wedged for garnish)
- ½ cup peanuts (crushed for garnish)

Method:
1. Mix ginger, garlic powder and the salt and pepper into a bowl.
2. Toss the chicken tenders in the mixture until they are coated.
3. Heat the peanut oil in a skillet over medium/high heat.
4. Once the oil gets hot, add the chicken and cook for about 3 minutes. Turn only once and cook until they are done all the way through.
5. Remove chicken when done and cut into quarter-inch slices. Set it aside.
6. Scramble eggs in the skillet for about a minute, then remove them and set them aside.
7. Reduce the heat to medium-low and add the broth, peanut butter, tamari, scallion, pepper flakes, garlic, and vinegar. Then cook for three minutes and stir well.
8. Add chicken, eggs, zucchini noodles and sprouts. Toss to coat and cook for a minute.
9. Sever the pad Thai with a garnish of lime wedges and peanuts.

Quick 'N Easy Buffalo Wings

Cook Time: 30 minutes
Servings: 2

Ingredients:
- 6 chicken wings
- ½ cup red hot sauce
- Salt and pepper, to taste
- Garlic powder, to taste
- 1 tsp paprika
- 2 tbsp butter
- 1 tsp cayenne (optional)

Method:
1. Break chicken wings into to pieces, then pour a little bit of red hot sauce over, just enough to coat them lightly.
2. Put the desired seasonings on your wings and toss to ensure they are coated well.
3. Put them in a refrigerator for an hour (If you are in a bind for time, you can skip this step).
4. Turn the broiler on so it can warm up. Use foil to line a baking sheet. Place the chicken wings on the sheet with some space between them. Place the oven rack close to the broiler.
5. Let the chicken wings cook under the broiler for 8 minutes. The tops should start to turn brown.
6. While the wings are cooking, melt the butter and the rest of the hot sauce in a pan. Add a little cayenne pepper for spicier wings.
7. Once the butter is completely melted, remove it from the heat.
8. Flip the wings and broil them for another 6 to 8 minutes watching them closely.
9. After the wings are browned on each side, place them in a deep bowl and pour the hot sauce over them. Toss them to coat evenly. Enjoy!

Chicken Curry

Cook Time: Approximately 1 hour
Servings: 8

Ingredients:
- 2 tbsp olive oil, butter or coconut oil
- 8 boneless chicken thighs, cut into 1-inch pieces
- 1 large onion, cut into pieces
- 3 small zucchini, sliced
- 1 tsp minced garlic
- 1 tbsp curry powder
- ½ tsp paprika
- 2 tsp salt
- 2 15-oz. cans coconut milk
- 1 cup of tomatoes
- Cilantro (garnish)

Method:
1. Heat oil in a pot on high heat, then add the chicken and cook until all the pieces are browned on both sides.
2. Remove chicken from oil and set aside, but leave the oil in the pan.
3. Sauté the onion and zucchini until they are lightly browned.
4. Add other spices (garlic, curry, paprika and salt) and sauté for only 30 seconds.
5. Add chicken and coconut milk in the pan and bring all of it to a boil.
6. Reduce heat and simmer, covered for about 30 minutes. Chicken should be tender.
7. Once the chicken is done, add tomatoes to the pot and cook for 5 more minutes.
8. Serve in a bowl like a soup and garnish with cilantro.

Chicken Stew – Crockpot Style

Cook Time: About 2 hours
Servings: 4

Ingredients:
- 2 cups chicken stock
- 2 sticks celery, diced
- 1 onion, diced
- 28 oz. chicken, diced into one-inch pieces
- ½ tsp rosemary
- 3 garlic cloves, minced
- ¼ tsp thyme
- ½ tsp oregano
- 2 carrots (optional if you want to reduce carbs)
- Salt and pepper, to taste
- ½ cup cream
- 1 cup fresh spinach leaves
- Xanthan gum for thickness (about 1/8 tsp)

Method:
1. Put chicken stock, celery, onion, chicken, spices and carrots (optional) into a crock pot that is at least a 3-quart capacity. Cook on high for two hours or on low for four.
2. Add salt and pepper as desired.
3. Stir in the heavy cream and spinach leaves.
4. Thicken soup with xanthan gum to the thickness you desire. Start with 1/8 teaspoon and add more if desired.
5. Continue to stir and cook for at least 10 more minutes.

Chicken Enchilada Keto-Style

Cook Time: 30 minutes
Servings: 4 to 6

Ingredients:
- 2 to 3 chicken breasts
- ¾ red enchilada sauce
- 1 can of green chilies (4 oz.)
- ¼ cup onions
- ¼ cup water
- Seasonings to taste
- 12-oz. bag of steam-able cauliflower rice
- Toppings of choice (avocado, cheese, Roma tomatoes, jalapeno)

Method:
1. Cook chicken breasts in a skillet on medium heat. Cook them until they are lightly browned. Cutting each breast into 3 or 4 pieces helps them cook faster.
2. Add enchilada sauce, chilies, onions, and water. Cover, and reduce heat to a simmer. Continue to cook until the chicken is completely done.
3. Take out the chicken from the skillet and shred it using forks, then add it back to the sauce and allow it to simmer for 10 minutes while uncovered. Most of the liquid will be soaked up.
4. Prepare cauliflower rice per the instructions on the bag.
5. Chop up your preferred toppings.
6. Top cauliflower rice with chicken, cheese and preferred toppings.

Easy Lemon Fried Chicken

Cook Time: 20 Minutes
Servings: 1

Ingredients:
- 1 chicken breast
- Lemon zest and juice
- 1 to 2 tsp of avocado oil or olive oil
- ¼ tsp salt
- 1/8 tsp black pepper

Method:
1. Place all ingredients in a zipper bag, pressing the bag to remove all the air. Zip and seal.
2. Using a rolling pin or a meat pounder, flatten the chicken into an even thickness.
3. Marinate for 30 minutes for the absolute best results, however, you can cook it immediately.
4. Place a skillet on medium-high heat and add your choice of oil.
5. Cook each side of the chicken for about 4 to 5 minutes – or until it is cooked all the way through.
6. Remove from heat and let chicken rest for about 5 minutes before slicing it.

Spinach-Stuffed Chicken

Cook Time: 45 minutes
Servings: 6

Ingredients:
- 6 chicken fillets or breasts
- 6 tbsp cream cheese
- 2 slices of bacon, diced
- A handful of fresh spinach
- Olive oil

Method:
1. Slice chicken breasts down the middle, without cutting them all the way through. You are making a "pocket."
2. Place some cream cheese, bacon and some chopped spinach in the middle of each fillet.
3. Fold the breast over and place a toothpick to hold it closed and keep the filling inside.
4. Place the stuffed chicken breasts in an oiled baking pan and pour a little oil over the tops of them.
5. Bake at 350 degrees (F) in the oven for 30 minutes or until the center is fully cooked. Cooking times can vary depends on the size of the chicken fillets and their thickness.

Chicken Kiev

Cook Time: 50 minutes
Servings: 2

Ingredients:
- 2 6-oz. chicken breasts
- Salt and pepper, to taste
- Parsley
- Tarragon
- 4 tbsp butter
- 1 green onion
- 2 garlic cloves
- 1 oz. of pork rinds
- 1 egg
- ¼ cup coconut flour

Method:
1. Pound chicken breasts until they are about ½-inch thick. Season with salt, pepper, parsley and tarragon to taste.
2. Put tabs of butter on each piece of chicken, then sprinkle with chopped green onion and garlic.
3. Roll the chicken up and hold it in place using toothpicks.
4. Prepare the "bread crumbs" by crushing pork rinds in a processor or Nutri-bullet.
5. Place the crumbled pork rinds in a bowl. Then scramble the egg in another bowl and place the coconut flour in a third bowl.
6. Coat each piece of chicken with the coconut flour first, making sure all sides are sealed. Then dip the chicken in the beaten egg and then coat it with the pork rinds.
7. Set the coated chicken in the fridge for about half an hour.
8. Preheat oven to 350 degrees (F).
9. Put chicken pieces in a hot, well-oiled skillet, and fry them on all sides.
10. Place the chicken in a baking dish and put it in the oven to bake for 20 minutes. Baste the chicken with any butter that seeps out.
11. Serve chicken on a bed of arugula.

Chicken Chili

Cook Time: 30 minutes
Servings: 6

Ingredients:
- 4 large chicken breasts
- 1 tbsp butter
- ½ chopped onion
- 2 cups chicken broth
- 10-oz. can of tomatoes
- 2 oz. tomato paste
- 1 tbsp chili powder
- 1 tbsp cumin
- ½ tbsp garlic powder
- 1 seeded and chopped jalapeno (optional)
- 4 oz. cream cheese
- Salt and pepper, to taste

Method:
1. Start by boiling the chicken breasts in water or in broth for about 10 minutes. They need to be barely covered by liquid.
2. As soon as the pink is gone from the meat, remove the chicken from the liquid and shred them using forks.
3. Using a large stockpot, melt the butter then add the onions and cook them until they are translucent.
4. Add in the shredded chicken, broth, tomatoes, tomato paste and the spices. Add jalapeno if desired.
5. Gently stir the ingredients while heating to a boil.
6. Once the pot is boiling, cover the pot and reduce the heat and simmer over medium-low heat for about 10 minutes.
7. Cut the cream cheese into 1-inch cubes.
8. Add the cream cheese to the pot and turn the heat to medium-high. Continue stirring until all the cream cheese is blended in.
9. Remove from heat. Add salt and pepper to taste preferences.
10. Enjoy! You may also enjoy garnishing with different toppings such as cilantro or Monterey Jack cheese.

Creamy Tuscan Chicken

Cook Time: About 30 minutes
Servings: 4 to 6

Ingredients:

- 2 tbsp olive oil
- 1 ½ lb. boneless chicken sliced thinly
- 1 cup of heavy cream
- ½ cup chicken broth
- 1 tsp garlic powder
- 1 tsp Italian seasonings
- ½ cup Parmesan cheese
- 1 cup fresh chopped spinach
- ½ cup sun-dried tomatoes

Method:

1. Add olive oil and chicken to a skillet over medium-high heat. Cook each side of the chicken for 3 to 5 minutes, or until they are brown and there's no pink in the middle. Remove the chicken and set it aside.
2. Whisk together the cream, broth, garlic powder, Italian herbs and Parmesan cheese over a medium heat. Gently stir until the mixture begins to thicken.
3. Add the spinach and tomatoes. Simmer just until the spinach wilts. Then add the chicken back into the sauce, stir well and enjoy

Bacon-Ranch Chicken Casserole

Cook Time: 45 minutes
Serves: 2

Ingredients:
- 8 oz. package of cream cheese
- 4 oz. sour cream
- 4 oz. Keto-approved mayonnaise
- ½ tbsp dill
- 1 tbsp Parsley
- ½ tbsp garlic powder
- ½ tsp salt
- ½ tsp pepper
- 1 ½ lb. cooked, cubed chicken
- 1 onion, minced
- 1 to 1 ½ cups of veggies (choose from broccoli, cauliflower or spinach)
- 8 oz. cheddar cheese (shredded)
- ¼ cup plus 2 tbsp bacon crumbles

Method:
1. Preheat oven to 350 degrees (F).
2. Use a large bowl and combine the cream cheese, sour cream, Keto mayo, and the spices. Mix them together thoroughly.
3. Once mixed well, add the chicken, onion, vegetable of choice, ¾ of the cheese and ¼ cup of the bacon. Mix well.
4. Oil a 9X13 baking dish and put the mixture into the dish.
5. Sprinkle the rest of the cheese and bacon bits on the top.
6. Bake for about 35 minutes, just until hot. Enjoy!

Leftover Turkey (or Chicken) Casserole

Cook Time: 45 minutes
Servings: 4-5

Ingredients:
- 2 tbsp unsalted butter
- 1 medium onion, chopped
- 2 stalks of celery, chopped
- 1 to 2 jalapeno peppers, chopped
- 1 large garlic clove, minced
- 8 oz. cream cheese
- ½ cup cream
- 1 tsp Worcestershire sauce
- ¼ tsp salt
- ¼ tsp pepper
- 2 cups leftover chicken or turkey, chopped
- 6 oz. cheddar cheese
- 2 scallions, sliced thinly (garnish)

Method:
1. Grease a 1 ½ quart casserole dish.
2. Melt 2 tablespoons of butter over medium heat.
3. As soon as it is melted, add onion and celery. Cook, stirring occasionally, until they are soft, but not browned. This takes about 8 minutes.
4. Reduce heat to low and add the jalapeno and garlic. Cook for about a minute, then stir in the cream cheese, cream, Worcestershire, salt and pepper. Whisk until these ingredients are combined.
5. Pour the cream and cheese mixture into a bowl, then stir in the chicken (or turkey) and ¾ of the cheddar cheese.
6. After it is well mixed, pour it all into the casserole dish then sprinkle the rest of the cheddar cheese on top.
7. Cook in the oven for 20 to 25 minutes, then turn the broiler on and brown the top for a few seconds.
8. Sprinkle scallions on top and serve.

Chicken Pot Pie

Cook Time: approximately 1 hour
Servings: 8

Ingredients:

Chicken Pie Filling:
- 1 tbsp butter
- 1 ½ lb. chicken breasts (cut into ½-inch cubes)
- 4 oz. chopped yellow onion
- ¼ cup finely diced carrots
- Sea salt and black pepper, to taste
- 1 crushed clove of garlic
- ½ tsp dried thyme
- 1 tbsp white wine vinegar
- 1 cup chicken broth
- ½ cup heavy cream
- ¼ cup green peas

Chicken Pot Pie Topping:
- 1 cup fine almond flour
- 1 tbsp ground flax seeds
- ½ tsp xanthan gum
- ¼ tsp sea salt
- 1 tsp baking powder
- 2 tbsp butter (cut into two pieces)
- 1 egg white
- 2 tbsp sour cream

Method:
1. Preheat oven to 400 degrees (F) and grease a 9-inch round baking pan.
2. Melt butter in a skillet over medium high heat.
3. Once the butter is melted, put the diced chicken in the butter. Fry until the sides are browned, but not completely cooked.
4. Add onion and carrots to the skillet. Sprinkle with a little salt and pepper, then turn the heat down to medium-low. Continue cooking, stirring occasionally until onions are browned on the edges but not quite tender.
5. Stir in the garlic and the thyme. Cook for one minute stirring constantly.

6. Stir in the vinegar and cook until it is almost totally evaporated, then pour in the broth.
7. Simmer broth on medium-high heat stirring occasionally. Let it cook for 15 to 20 minutes or until it thickens.
8. After the broth has thickened up, add the cream and peas.
9. Bring the mixture back to a simmer and reduce to low heat setting. Simmer until the mixture has thickened and is a gravy consistency. Taste then season with salt and pepper as desired.
10. Whisk the almond flour, flax seeds, xanthan gum, baking powder and salt together in a bowl.
11. Cut the butter into the dry ingredients until it is mealy.
12. Whisk the egg white and sour cream together in a small bowl and then stir it into the dry ingredients.
13. Roll it into a ball and then press it out into an 8-inch circle on a piece of parchment paper.
14. To assemble, pour the chicken filling into the greased baking dish. Gently place the dough over the filling.
15. Bake it in the oven for 10 to 12 minutes or until the topping is nicely browned.

Chicken "n Cream with Poblano Peppers

Cook Time: About 30 minutes
Servings: 4

Ingredients:
- 2 roasted Poblano peppers
- 1 ¼ lb. chicken fillets
- 1 tbsp olive oil
- Salt and pepper, to taste
- 3 ½ oz. sliced onion
- 1 large garlic clove
- ¼ cup dry white wine
- 1 cup of heavy cream
- 1/8 tsp cumin

Method:
1. Prepare peppers by roasting them until the sides are blackened. They can be roasted over a gas burner or in a broiler. Once they are roasted, steam and peel then refrigerate until you need them.
2. Set the chicken out for 20 minutes so it can be close to room temperature.
3. Put teaspoons of olive oil in a non-stick or stainless-steel skillet (Do not use cast iron).
4. Dry the chicken off by blotting with a towel then massage the rest of the oil on the chicken and season with salt and pepper as desired.
5. Once the pan with oil is hot, cook the chicken fillets for 4 to 6 minutes on each side. Remove chicken and set aside.
6. Make the sauce by sautéing the onions and garlic for a minute over medium heat. Remove the pan from the heat to add the dry wine.
7. Place it back on the heat and cook until the wine evaporates.
8. Add cream, poblano peppers and cumin. Cook the sauce until it thickens to the desired consistency. Remember it thickens more as it cools. Taste the sauce and add salt and pepper to taste.
9. Pour the sauce over the chicken.

Turkey Meatballs and Kale Soup

Cook Time: 30 minutes
Servings: 4 to 6

Ingredients:

For the Meatballs:
- 1 lb. of ground turkey
- 1 egg
- 2 to 4 tbsp almond flour (or coconut)
- 2 cloves of crushed garlic (or ¼ tsp garlic powder)
- ¾ tsp salt
- Black pepper, to taste
- 2 tbsp fresh herbs or ½ tsp dried herbs (dill, cilantro, basil, parsley)
- 2 tbsp butter, coconut oil or ghee

For the Soup:
- 2 tbsp butter, coconut oil or ghee
- 1 onion, diced
- 4 chipped carrots (or less to cut carbs)
- 2 garlic cloves, diced
- 2 bay leaves
- 6 cups chicken or vegetable broth
- Bunch of kale (de-stemmed and chopped)

Garnish:
- Fresh herbs – parsley, dill, cilantro, basil
- Red pepper flakes

Method:

1. Make the meatballs by combining the turkey, egg, flour, garlic, salt and pepper, and herbs all together.
2. Once it is mixed well, form it into 1 ½ inch balls. It should make about 25 meatballs.
3. Heat 2 Tablespoons of oil in a large skillet over a medium high heat.
4. Add meatballs and cook them for about 3 to 4 minutes, making sure all sides are browned. It may take more than one batch. Once they are done, set them aside.
5. Make the soup by heating 2 tablespoons of fat in a large soup pot.
6. Add in the onions, carrots and garlic. Cook in the oil until the onions are translucent. This will take about 5 minutes.

7. Add bay leaves, broth and the meatballs.
8. Bring the soup to a boil then, reduce heat to a simmer. Simmer for about 5 minutes.
9. Add the de-stemmed and chopped kale and continue cooking until the meatballs are fully cooked. This should take about 5 to 7 minutes.
10. Add garnish of fresh herbs and pepper flakes and serve.

Chicken Zucchini Pasta with Pistachios

Cook Time: 40 minutes
Serves: 2 to 4

Ingredients:
Noodles:
- 2 to 2.5 lb. zucchini
- 1 tbsp salt
- 1 tbsp olive oil
- 2 garlic cloves
- ¼ tsp cumin
- ¼ tsp black pepper

Chicken:
- 4 boneless chicken breasts (4 to 6 ounces each)
- 1 tbsp olive oil or ghee
- Salt and black pepper, to taste

Aromatics:
- 2 Scallions
- 7 to 10 leaves of fresh mint
- ¼ cup pistachios (shelled)
- 1 tbsp lemon juice

Method:
1. Use a spiralizer to create zucchini noodles. Place the noodles in a colander and toss with salt so the strands are lightly coated with salt. Put the colander in the sink and let it drain.
2. Pound the chicken breasts until they are about ½ inch thick.
3. Slice each chicken breast crosswise into strips.
4. Place the tablespoon of oil or ghee in a skillet and heat for 2 to 3 minutes over medium-high heat.
5. Place the chicken strips in the hot oil and sprinkle them with salt and pepper to taste. Turn the chicken strips to cover them in oil.
6. Spread the chicken strips over the bottom of the skillet in a single layer. Let them cook for 2 to 3 minutes, then turn and cook 2 to 3 minutes on the other side. Keep flipping and cooking the chicken until it is browned well on most sides. This may take about 2 more minutes.

7. Once the chicken is browned well, remove from the skillet and place on a plate. Cover it loosely with a piece of foil.
8. Prep the aromatics by slicing the scallions, mincing the mint leaves and chopping the pistachios. Add all these ingredients to a bowl and mix in the lemon juice with a fork. Set aside.
9. To cook the noodles, place the oil in a small bowl.
10. Peel, then crush the cloves of garlic, and add it to the garlic in the bowl. Mix with a fork and set aside.
11. Rinse and drain the zucchini noodles and squeeze them in a towel to remove extra water.
12. Re-heat the skillet and oil used for the chicken, and sauté the noodles over medium-high heat for 2 to 3 minutes.
13. Push the noodles over to one side of the pan and reduce heat to medium low. Add the garlic and stir. Cook for just 20 seconds, continuing to stir.
14. Stir the noodles into the oil until they are coated. Turn the heat off, and add the chicken and the mint mixture.

ıg

le of the baking

ı down. Roasting time
e, approximately 8 minutes ı

callions to serve.

Seafood

Pan-Roasted Salmon with Red Cabbage

Cook Time: Less than an hour
Serves: 4

Ingredients:

- 4 6-oz. salmon fillets (or other type of fish) 1-inch thick and patted dry
- 3 tbsp avocado oil or EVVO plus just a bit more to coat fillets
- 8 chopped scallions
- Shredded head of red cabbage (small to medium)
- ¼ cup fresh parsley finely chopped

Method:

1. Preheat oven to 425 degrees (F).
2. Rub salmon with oil of choice and season to taste preference with salt and pepper. Then set aside.
3. Save a little bit of the scallions for a garnish and toss the rest with the cabbage and oil. Season with salt and pepper.
4. Spread the cabbage and scallions on a rimmed baking sheet (18X13) and cook for 25 minutes.
5. Stir the scallions and cabbage and push to the outsi   sheet, and lay the fillets in the center.
   (Make sure the salmon is placed on the pan ski   varies depending on how thick the fish or salmon fillets aι   for each inch is good.)
6. Top baked salmon with parsley and the rest of the sι

Seafood

Pan-Roasted Salmon with Red Cabbage

Cook Time: Less than an hour
Serves: 4

Ingredients:
- 4 6-oz. salmon fillets (or other type of fish) 1-inch thick and patted dry
- 3 tbsp avocado oil or EVVO plus just a bit more to coat fillets
- 8 chopped scallions
- Shredded head of red cabbage (small to medium)
- ¼ cup fresh parsley finely chopped

Method:
1. Preheat oven to 425 degrees (F).
2. Rub salmon with oil of choice and season to taste preference with salt and pepper. Then set aside.
3. Save a little bit of the scallions for a garnish and toss the rest with the cabbage and oil. Season with salt and pepper.
4. Spread the cabbage and scallions on a rimmed baking sheet (18X13) and cook for 25 minutes.
5. Stir the scallions and cabbage and push to the outside of the baking sheet, and lay the fillets in the center.
   (Make sure the salmon is placed on the pan skin down. Roasting time varies depending on how thick the fish or salmon fillets are, approximately 8 minutes for each inch is good.)
6. Top baked salmon with parsley and the rest of the scallions to serve.

7. Once the chicken is browned well, remove from the skillet and place on a plate. Cover it loosely with a piece of foil.
8. Prep the aromatics by slicing the scallions, mincing the mint leaves and chopping the pistachios. Add all these ingredients to a bowl and mix in the lemon juice with a fork. Set aside.
9. To cook the noodles, place the oil in a small bowl.
10. Peel, then crush the cloves of garlic, and add it to the garlic in the bowl. Mix with a fork and set aside.
11. Rinse and drain the zucchini noodles and squeeze them in a towel to remove extra water.
12. Re-heat the skillet and oil used for the chicken, and sauté the noodles over medium-high heat for 2 to 3 minutes.
13. Push the noodles over to one side of the pan and reduce heat to medium low. Add the garlic and stir. Cook for just 20 seconds, continuing to stir.
14. Stir the noodles into the oil until they are coated. Turn the heat off, and add the chicken and the mint mixture.

Watercress & Herb Sauce with Fish

Cook Time: About 30 minutes
Servings: 2

Ingredients:
- 2 6-oz. skinless white fish about 1 to 1½ inch thick (halibut is preferred)
- Can of coconut milk (13.5 oz.)
- 2 cloves of garlic finely chopped
- 1 cup of cilantro leaves
- 1 tbsp ginger – finely chopped
- 1 ½ cups watercress leaves
- ¼ cup green onion tops chopped
- ¼ tsp kosher salt
- Fresh herbs for garnish (parsley, cilantro, basil)
- Lime wedge (garnish)

Method:
1. Salt the fish lightly then set it aside.
2. Create a green sauce by combining coconut milk, garlic, cilantro, ginger, watercress, green onions, and salt with a blender. Blend until you have a smooth sauce.
3. Pour the green sauce into a skillet and simmer.
4. Add the fish and then cover. Time varies based on thickness of the fish, but it should only take between 5 to 7 minutes.
5. Serve as a stand-alone dish or over sautéed spinach or cauliflower rice.

Fish Chowder

Cook Time: Less than an hour
Servings: 8

Ingredients:
- 5 slices of bacon chopped
- 4 tbsp butter
- 1 yellow onion, diced
- 4 cloves of garlic, minced
- ¼ cup white wine
- 1 tsp paprika
- 1 tsp thyme
- 3 cups chicken stock
- 1 head of cauliflower
- 2 cups cream
- 1 lb. white fish (halibut or cod)
- 1 tsp lemon juice
- 1 tsp tabasco
- Salt and pepper, to taste
- ½ cup shredded sharp cheddar cheese
- 1 cup grated Parmesan cheese

Method:
1. Cook the bacon in a soup pot for about 10 minutes on low heat. Stir it often so the bacon is crisp and the fat renders.
2. Add the butter and chopped onion and turn heat up to medium-high. Continue to cook for about 5 minutes, then add garlic and cook 5 more minutes until the onion softens.
3. Add white wine to deglaze and stir for one full minute.
4. Then add the paprika, thyme, and chicken stock.
5. Add the chopped cauliflower. Bring pot to a boil and then reduce to a simmer and let it cook for 20 to 25 minutes or until the cauliflower is soft.
6. Then add in the heavy cream and cook for 10 more minutes.
7. Blend the soup in a blender or using a handheld blender then return the soup to a low heat.
8. Add the rest of the ingredients and the cooked, shredded fish.
9. Add salt and pepper or other spices as desired.
10. Thicken the chowder with cheese, or let it cook down. If it gets too thick, use stock or cream to thin the liquid base.

Halibut with Parmesan Crust

Cook Time: About 30 minutes
Servings: 6

Ingredients:
- 6 halibut filets (about 1 to 2 lb.)
- 1 stick of butter (room temperature)
- 1 tbsp panko bread crumbs
- 1 tsp kosher salt
- ½ tsp black pepper
- 2 tsp garlic powder
- 1 tbsp parsley
- 3 tbsp grated Parmesan cheese

Method:
1. Preheat oven to 400 degrees (F).
2. Mix all ingredients in a bowl except the fish.
3. Pat halibut with a paper towel to dry and then lay the pieces on a greased baking sheet.
4. Carefully spread the Parmesan cheese mixture over the fish so that each piece is covered.
5. Bake fish for 10 to 12 minutes rotating the pan half way through.
6. Move fish to the broiler for 2 to 3 minutes to brown the top.

Lemon-Garlic Shrimp

Cook Time: 20 minutes
Servings: 2

Ingredients:
- 2 tbsp ghee
- 8 garlic cloves, minced
- ½ tbsp lemon juice
- ¼ tsp salt and black peper
- 1 lb. peeled and deveined shrimp
- 2 bell peppers, chopped
- 4 mushrooms
- 1 zucchini, chopped

Method:
1. Preheat oven to 400 degrees (F).
2. Melt ghee in a small pan and add the garlic, lemon juice, and pepper and salt.
3. Divide this mixture in half.
4. Using half the mixture, dip each shrimp in it and place them on skewers.
5. Place zucchini slices, mushrooms and pepper pieces on skewers.
6. Put the filled skewers on a baking tray and bake in the oven. Turn to bake about 5 minutes on each side.
7. Serve with the other half of the ghee-garlic mixture.

Creamy Fish Casserole

Cook Time: 40 minutes
Servings: 4

Ingredients:
- 1 lb. broccoli (substitute spinach for fewer carbs)
- 2 tbsp olive oil
- Salt and pepper, to taste
- 6 scallions
- 2 tbsp small capers
- Butter to grease the casserole dish
- 1.5 lb. white fish
- 1 tbsp parsley
- 1 ¼ cups whipping cream
- 1 tbsp Dijon mustard
- 3 oz. butter
- 5+ oz. leafy greens

Method:
1. Preheat oven to 400 degrees (F).
2. Divide broccoli out into small florets and keep the stems. Use a potato peeler to peel the stems if they are tough.
3. Fry broccoli in oil for 5 minutes on medium heat until florets are soft. Add salt and pepper.
4. Add chopped scallions and capers then fry for another 1 to 2 minutes.
5. Place the fried vegetables in the greased baking dish.
6. Lay the fish fillets in amongst the veggies.
7. Mix parsley, cream and mustard with a whisk and then pour the mixture over the fish and vegetables. Add a few tabs of butter to the top.
8. Bake 20 minutes or until the fish is done, and serve with your choice of greens. It should flake easily with a fork.

Salmon/Avocado Salsa

Cook Time: About 25 minutes
Servings: 4 to 6

Ingredients:
- 2 lb. salmon fillets
- 1 tsp cumin
- 1 tsp smoked paprika
- 1 tsp onion powder
- Salt and pepper, to taste
- 1 to 2 tbsp oil (butter, avocado oil, olive oil, coconut oil)

Ingredients for Avocado Salsa:
- 2 peeled and diced avocados
- 1 small red onion, diced
- 3 peppers, seeded and diced (jalapeno, banana)
- Juice from 3 limes
- 2 tbsp olive oil
- 2 tbsp freshly chopped cilantro
- Salt and pepper, to personal taste

Method:
1. Combine all the ingredients for the avocado salsa in a bowl. Set it in the fridge while you prepare the salmon.
2. Preheat the oven to 400 degrees (F).
3. Lightly grease a baking pan and then place the salmon fillets in the pan.
4. Combine cumin, paprika, onion powder, salt and pepper in a bowl. Then rub the prepared spices over each piece of salmon.
5. Place a small tab of butter on each fillet.
6. Bake salmon for 12 to 15 minutes or until the salmon flakes easily.
7. Take out the avocado salsa and serve alongside the salmon.

Tuna Fish Patties

Cook Time: 20 minutes
Servings: 2

Ingredients:
- 2 5 or 6 oz. cans tuna or salmon
- 1 tbsp freshly chopped basil
- 1 jalapeno pepperdiced)
- 2 eggs
- 2 tbsp coconut flour
- 2 tbsp coconut flakes
- 2 tbsp olive oil
- ½ tsp salt
- 1 tbsp coconut oil (for cooking)

Method:
1. Take the tuna from the can and use a fork to flake it.
2. Mix all the ingredients together in a single bowl, including the tuna.
3. Make 4 patties from the mixture.
4. Heat one tablespoon of coconut oil in a skillet over medium-high heat.
5. Place the four patties in the heated oil and cook until they are golden brown on one side.
6. Turn the patties over and cook them until the other side is golden.

Salmon Cucumber Wraps

Cook Time: 5 minutes
Servings: 2

Ingredients:
- 1 tbsp coconut cream
- 4 thin slices of ham
- 3.5 oz. smoked salmon
- ½ cucumber sliced thinly
- Leafy green salad

Method:
1. Spread a little coconut cream on each ham slice.
2. Place a slice of smoked salmon on top of the coconut cream on each ham slice.
3. Place a thin slice of cucumber on top of each piece of salmon.
4. Roll up the wrap and serve with a leafy green salad.

Quick 'n Easy Shrimp Scampi

Cook Time: 15 minutes
Servings: 2

Ingredients:
- 2 tbsp olive oil
- 2 tbsp butter
- 1 clove garlics, sliced
- ½ cup dry white wine
- ½ tsp salt
- 1/8 tsp pepper
- 2 lb. extra-large shrimps, peeled and deveined
- 1/3 cup fresh chopped parsley
- 2 tbsp lemon juice
- 1 tsp lemon zest
- ¼ tsp red pepper flakes (optional)
- 3 cups cooked spaghetti squash
- Parmesan cheese for garnish (optional)

Method:
1. Heat the oil and butter in a skillet.
2. Add garlic and cook for 2 to 3 minutes or until fragrant.
3. Add wine, salt, red and black pepper and cook for 2 more minutes.
4. Add shrimp and cook 2 to 3 minutes longer – just until the shrimp is opaque.
5. Remove from heat and then add parsley, lemon juice, lemon zest and pepper flakes and toss.
6. Serve over spaghetti squash and garnish with Parmesan cheese.

Keto Fish Nuggets

Cook Time: 30 minutes
Servings: 3

Ingredients:
- 3 frozen tilapia fillets
- ½ cup ground pork rinds
- ½ cup Parmesan cheese
- Salt, pepper, garlic powder, cayenne – any seasonings you like
- 1 egg
- 1 tbsp cream
- 3 tbsp of olive oil

Method:
1. Let the fish thaw by putting the packaged fish in hot water for a few minutes.
2. Grind pork rinds into a powder using a food processor. They need to be ground or they will not stick to the fish.
3. Mix the pork rind, Parmesan and whatever spices you prefer together in a bowl.
4. In another bowl, whisk together the egg and cream.
5. Cut the fish fillets into 1-inch squares. Making them smaller will help them cook faster and will help keep the "breading" from burning.
6. Heat a skillet over a medium-high heat and add just enough oil to coat the surface with about ¼ inch of oil.
7. Coat the fish nuggets with the egg mixture.
8. Then coated them well with the pork rind and cheese mixture, then toss them in the oil.
9. Fry nuggets until they are golden brown, usually about 2 to 3 minutes.
10. Flip the nuggets half way through to brown on both sides.

Spicy Fish Stew

Cook Time: 30 minutes
Servings: 2

Ingredients:
- 1 lb. wild-caught white fish
- 1 juiced lime
- 1 jalapeno pepper
- ½ tbsp. olive oil
- 1 red pepper
- 1 yellow pepper
- 1 medium onion
- 2 garlic cloves, minced
- 1 tsp paprika
- 1 tsp salt
- ¼ tsp black pepper
- 2 cups chicken bone broth
- 2 cups chopped tomatoes
- 15 oz. coconut milk
- Cilantro/extra lime wedges for garnish

Method:
1. Place fish in a large non-reactive bowl. Add the lime juice and let it marinate while you work on the rest of the recipe.
2. Heat the olive oil in a large pan.
3. Once the oil is hot, sauté peppers and onions until the onions are translucent. This should take 3 to 4 minutes.
4. Then add the garlic and sauté for an additional 30 seconds.
5. Add the other spices, broth and tomatoes. Stir well and bring the mixture to a boil.
6. Then add the marinating fish and coconut milk. Stir well and bring to a boil.
7. Cover and reduce the heat to medium-low and simmer until the fish is flakey. This should take about 10 minutes.
8. Remove the cover, sprinkle the cilantro on the fish and serve with extra lime wedges.

One-Pan Lemon, Butter, Garlic Shrimp with Asparagus

Cook Time: 25 minutes
Servings: 4 to 6

Ingredients:

Asparagus
- 1 lb. of asparagus
- 1 tbsp olive oil
- 1 clove of garlic, minced
- ¼ tsp salt
- 1/8 tsp pepper

Shrimp
- 1 ½ lb. uncooked, peeled and deveined shrimp
- 1 tbsp olive oil
- 2 to 3 cloves of garlic
- ½ tsp salt
- ¼ tsp paprika
- 1/8 tsp pepper
- 1/8 to ¼ tsp red pepper flakes
- 3 tbsp chopped parsley
- 3 tbsp butter (cubed)
- 1 ½ tbsp lemon juice

Method:
1. Preheat oven to 400 degrees (F).
2. Use foil to line a jelly roll pan, lightly coat it with oil.
3. Place asparagus on one end and drizzle one tablespoon of olive oil over it.
4. Add garlic, salt and pepper. Toss the asparagus until it is evenly coated.
5. Lay it out on a single layer and roast it for 4 to 6 minutes.
6. Remove tails from the shrimp.
7. Remove the asparagus from the oven, and slide it all to one end of the pan keeping it all in a single layer.
8. Place the shrimp on the other end of the pan and drizzle it with a tablespoon of olive oil.
9. Add garlic, ½ teaspoon of salt, ¼ teaspoon of paprika, pepper, red chili flakes and parsley. Toss the shrimp until it is evenly coated and then lay them out in a single layer.

10. Place a cube of butter on the top of the asparagus. Put two cubes of butter on the shrimp.
11. Roast for about 6 minutes, or until the shrimp becomes opaque.
12. Remove from oven and drizzle shrimp with lemon juice. Add salt and pepper to taste and enjoy.

Shrimp and Sausage Skillet

Cook Time: 20 minutes
Servings: 4

Ingredients:
- Choice of oil (coconut or olive)
- 1 lb. shrimps, deveined and peeled (medium or large)
- 2 tsp Old Bay seasoning
- ½ cup yellow onion
- ¾ cup red bell pepper
- ¾ cup green bell pepper
- 1 zucchini
- 6 oz. of precooked sausage chopped
- 2 cloves of garlic, diced
- ¼ cup chicken stock
- Salt and pepper, to taste
- Pinch of red pepper flakes
- Parsley for a garnish

Method:
1. Heat your choice of oil in a large skillet over a medium high heat.
2. Season the shrimp with Old Bay seasoning.
3. Cook the shrimp for 3 to 4 minutes or until it is opaque in appearance. Then set it aside.
4. In the same skillet, add 2 tablespoons of oil and cook the onions and bell peppers for about 2 minutes.
5. Add chopped zucchini and sausage to the skillet and cook it for about 2 more minutes.
6. Place the cooked shrimp back into the skillet. Add the garlic and cook for about a minute.
7. Add the chicken stock and mix so everything is moistened.
8. Add salt, pepper and red pepper flakes to your taste preference.
9. Remove from heat and add parsley as a garnish.

Wasabi Salmon Burgers

Cook Time: 20 mins
Servings: 4

Ingredients:
- A 1 lb. salmon filet
- 1 tbsp fresh ginger, peeled and minced
- ¼ cup fresh scallions, chopped
- ¼ cup cilantro
- 2 eggs
- 1 tbsp lime Juice
- ½ cup blanched almond flour
- 1 tsp sea salt
- ¼ cup wasabi powder
- 1 tbsp water
- Coconut oil (for frying)

Method:
1. Rinse the salmon and pat it dry. Then cut it into quarter-inch cubes.
2. Combine salmon, ginger, scallions, cilantro, eggs, lime juice, almond flour and salt in a large mixing bowl.
3. In a smaller bowl, combine the wasabi powder and enough water to form a paste. Then add it to the salmon mixture.
4. Form salmon batter into 2-inch patties.
5. Heat oil in a skillet over medium-high heat. Sauté the patties until they are golden brown. This will take about 6 to 8 minutes on each side.

Appetizer

Cheddar Cheese Chips and Bacon Guacamole

Cook Time: 20 minutes
Serves: 4-6

Ingredients:
- 3 cups cheddar cheese, grated

For Guacamole:
- 2 strips of bacon, cooked then crumbled
- 1 tbsp lime zest
- 2 tbsp lime juice
- Small shallot, chopped finely
- Small clove of garlic, pressed
- 1 fresh jalapeno, chopped
- ¼ tsp salt
- 4 avocados

Method:
1. Preheat oven to 400 degrees (F) and line a baking sheet with parchment.
2. Drop grated cheddar cheese onto the parchment using a tablespoon. Mounds should be spaced out and you should be able to make around 16 mounds. Spread each mound out so they are circular.
3. Bake 8 minutes or until the cheese is bubbling and melted. Remember the cheese chips won't stay crispy for very long so prepare them right before making the guacamole.
4. Prepare all the ingredients for the guacamole. They should be ready, so they can be mixed with the avocadoes as soon as they are cut up.
5. Cut up the avocadoes then add the prepared ingredients. Use a fork to mash the guacamole mixture into the preferred texture.
6. Serve with cheddar cheese chips.

Low Carb Caprese Meatballs

Cook Time: approximately 30 minutes
Serves: 4-6

Ingredients:
- 1 lb. of ground turkey
- 1 medium egg
- ¼ cup almond flour
- ½ tsp salt
- ¼ tsp pepper
- ½ tsp garlic powder
- ½ cup shredded mozzarella cheese
- 2 tbsp chopped sun dried tomatoes
- 2 tbsp chopped fresh basil
- 2 tbsp olive oil (for frying)

Method:
1. Combine all the ingredients except for the olive oil in a bowl and mix them together. Then form the mixture into 16 meatballs.
2. Heat the olive oil in a large skillet and put the meatballs in the hot oil placing them about one inch apart.
3. Cook on low to medium heat for about 3 minutes per side or until they are thoroughly cooked. Be careful to not burn them as the cheese tends to melt out of the meatball a little bit. If they get dark too quickly, reduce the heat.
4. Serve meatballs alone as an appetizer or with marinara sauce. Or place meatballs on skewers with cherry tomatoes, basil leaves and fresh mozzarella.

Frittata and Tomatoes

Cook Time: 25 minutes
Servings: 2

Ingredients:
- ½ white onion
- 1 tbsp ghee
- 6 eggs
- Salt and fresh ground pepper, to taste
- 2 tbsp freshly chopped herbs (basil, chives)
-
- 2/3 cup crumbled soft cheese (feta works well)
- 2/3 cup cherry tomatoes

Method:
1. Preheat broiler or oven to 400 degrees (F).
2. Peel and slice the white onion.
3. Heat a small amount of ghee in a skillet and cook the sliced onions until they are lightly browned.
4. Crack all the eggs and add salt and pepper to taste. Add the chopped herbs.
5. Once the onion is brown, pour in the eggs and let it cook until the edges are opaque.
6. Add the crumbled cheese on the top and spread halved cherry tomatoes over the top.
7. Place it in the broiler (or oven) for 5 to 7 minutes or until the top is fully cooked.
8. Remove from the oven and serve!

Deviled Eggs with Avocado

Cook Time: Under 1 hour
Servings: 6

Ingredients:
- 4 to 6 eggs
- 1 medium avocado
- ¼ tsp sea salt
- ¼ tsp pepper
- ¼ tsp garlic powder
- ¼ tsp chili powder
- ¼ tsp cumin
- ¼ tsp smoked or regular paprika (optional)
- Lime juice
- 2 tbsp cilantro

Method:
1. Hard boil the eggs in a medium pot. Remove from heat and peel the eggs. Slice each egg lengthwise in half. Then remove the yolk.
2. Put the egg yolks and avocado in a bowl with the spices. Then mix them together until they are well combined.
3. Spoon the avocado with yolk mixture back into the empty egg halves.
4. Drizzle lime juice over the eggs and top with fresh cilantro for a tasty treat.

Cauliflower Grilled Cheese

Cook Time: Less than an hour
Servings: 4 slices of cauliflower "bread"

Ingredients:

- 1 medium head of raw cauliflower
- 1 large egg
- ½ cup Parmesan cheese, shredded
- 1 tsp Italian herb seasonings
- 2 slices white cheddar cheese

Method:

1. Preheat the oven to 450 degrees (F).
2. While it is heating, put the cauliflower in a food processor to pulse it until it's crumbs that are smaller than a rice granule.
3. Put cauliflower in a bowl and microwave it for two minutes. It should be soft.
4. Stir the cauliflower and put it back in the microwave for about five minutes. It should start to look dry.
5. Microwave for another 4-5 minutes. It should be moist to touch, but looks dry and clumped. *Cauliflower can be steamed for those who do not use the microwave.*
6. Allow the cauliflower to cool then add the egg, seasoning and Parmesan. Stir until the mixture forms a smooth paste.
7. Divide into four equal sized parts.
8. Put each on a baking sheet that has been lined with parchment or on a mat.
9. Press and shape the cauliflower into the shape of a slice of bread. They should be about ½ inch thick.
10. Bake for 15 to 18 minutes or until they turn a golden brown.
11. Remove from oven to cool.
12. Use a spatula to remove the cooled cauliflower from the parchment paper. Cauliflower bread is delicate, so it won't work to use a grill. Instead assemble the sandwiches by placing a slice of white cheddar cheese between two pieces of cauliflower bread.
13. Place the sandwiches in the oven, or a toaster oven and broil for 5 to 10 minutes. The cheese should melt, and the bread should be toasty.

Greek Avocado Salad

Cook Time: 10 minutes
Serves: 2

Ingredients:
Dressing:
- ¼ cup olive oil
- 2 tbsp red wine vinegar
- 1 large garlic clove
- 2 tsp dried oregano
- ¼ tsp salt

Salad:
- 1 large cucumber
- 4 vine ripe tomatoes
- 1 green bell pepper
- ½ red onion
- 7 oz. of feta cheese
- ½ cup pitted Kalamata olives
- 1 large avocado

Method:
1. Place all the ingredients for the dressing together and whisk.
2. Cut a cucumber in half lengthways and slice. Cut tomatoes into wedges. Deseed and slice a bell pepper, and chop up a red onion.
3. Mix all the fresh vegetables and other salad ingredients together

Onion Soup

Cook Time: 45 minutes to an hour
Servings: 6-8

Ingredients:
- 4 peeled and sliced onions
- 4 tbsp ghee
- Bone broth (2 cups chicken bone broth + 2 cups beef bone broth)
- 5 chopped garlic cloves
- Sea salt and pepper, to taste

Method:
1. Heat onions and ghee in a stock pot on medium heat and cook until the onions are slightly caramelized.
2. Add bone broth (all four cups) and garlic.
3. Season with salt and pepper.
4. Bring mixture to boiling and reduce heat to simmer. Simmer for 30 to 50 minutes. The longer the soup simmers, the more flavorful it will be.

Cucumber Bites

Cook Time: 15 minutes
Servings: About 4

Ingredients:
- 1 large cucumber or two small ones
- 1 avocado
- 3 to 4 oz. smoked salmon
- ½ tsp of white or black sesame seeds

Method:
1. Slice a cucumber into 1/4-inch thick rounds.
2. Slice an avocado, about the size of the cucumber rounds.
3. Place each avocado slice on each cucumber slice.
4. Cut salmon into slices that are about twice as long as the cucumber rounds. Fold the slice of salmon in half and put it on top of each avocado/cucumber.
5. Sprinkle the sesame seeds on the top.

Grilled Tomatoes and Apricot Jam

Cook Time: About 35 minutes
Servings: 6

Ingredients:
- 6 medium tomatoes
- 3 tsp apricot spread or sugar-free jam
- 2 tsp oregano
- Salt and pepper, to taste
- 3.5 oz. gouda cheese
- 1 tbsp olive oil
- 1.5 oz. watercress (garnish)
- Freshly ground black pepper (garnish)

Method:
1. Preheat the oven to 360 degrees (F).
2. Cut all the tomatoes in half. Place them on a lightly-greased baking tray.
3. Spread a small amount of apricot jam on each tomato half, then sprinkle oregano, salt and pepper to taste.
4. Sprinkle grated cheese and bake in the oven for 25 minutes.
5. Garnish with watercress, drizzle olive oil and top off with some black pepper.

Fried Green Beans

Cook Time: 20 minutes
Servings: 4

Ingredients:
- 12 oz. fresh green beans
- 2/3 grated Parmesan cheese
- ½ tsp sea salt or pink Himalayan salt
- ¼ tsp black pepper
- ½ tsp garlic powder
- ¼ tsp paprika
- 1 large egg

Method:
1. Preheat the oven to 400 degrees (F).
2. Snip the ends off the green beans, wash and dry.
3. Combine Parmesan cheese and seasonings on a plate and mix thoroughly. (Garlic powder and paprika are optional.)
4. Whisk the egg in a bowl. Drop the green beans into the egg so that it coats them, then press them gently into the Parmesan mixture by hand.
5. Place green beans on a greased baking sheet allowing plenty of room between the beans. Bake 10 minutes or until the cheese is slightly golden.
6. Let the green beans cool, then enjoy! They are good by themselves, or dipped in ranch or spicy mayo.

Kale Chips

Cook Time: 15 minutes
Serves: 2

Ingredients:
- 1 bunch of kale
- 2 tbsp olive oil
- ¼ cup nutritional yeast
- Sea salt

Method:
1. Preheat oven to 300 degrees (F) and place parchment paper on two baking pans or cookie sheets.
2. Wash the kale and pat dry using a paper towel. Remove the large stems from the kale. The spine can become extremely hard when baked.
3. Put the kale in a large bowl and toss with olive oil, yeast and salt.
4. Place the coated kale on the baking sheets. Do not layer them.
5. Bake for 10 to 15 minutes or until the leaves are crunchy and dry.

Coconut Chocolate Bars

Cook Time: About 45 minutes
Servings: 12

Ingredients:

Bottom Layer:
- 2 cups unsweetened coconut (shredded)
- 1/3 cup coconut oil
- 2 droppers of stevia

Chocolate Top Layer:
- 3 squares or 3 oz. of unsweetened chocolate
- 1 tbsp coconut oil
- 2 droppers of stevia (sweetener)

Method:

1. To make the bottom layer of the coconut bar, place the three ingredients for the bottom layer in a food processor. Use the S blade and process until it forms into dough.
2. Press the coconut dough into the bottom of a loaf pan (9X5), and put it in the freezer while you make the top layer.
3. Melt the chocolate and coconut oil using a double boiler or in the microwave. Stir in the sweetener.
4. Spread the topping over the frozen bottom layer and put it back in the freezer for about 30 minutes.
5. Remove from freezer and turn it upside down to take out from the loaf pan. Cut into 12 "bars." Store any remaining bars in the freezer.

Deviled Eggs with Bacon

Cook Time: 20 minutes
Serves: 2

Ingredients:
- 2 slices of bacon
- 5 hard boiled eggs
- ¼ cup keto mayonnaise
- 1 tsp Dijon mustard
- ¼ tsp cayenne pepper
- 1 tbsp bacon fat
- ½ tsp rosemary

Method:
1. Place two thin slices of bacon in a pan and fry on medium heat.
2. Remove cooked bacon and place on a paper towel. Cut or break the slices into pieces. Leave as much bacon grease in the pan as you can.
3. Cut the hard-boiled eggs in half and scoop out the yolks into a bowl.
4. Add mayo, Dijon mustard, cayenne, bacon fat and half the rosemary to the yolks and mix thoroughly.
5. Place some little bacon pieces in the hole left in the eggs. Then add the yolk mixture on top of the bacon bits, filling up the center of the eggs. Add the rest of the rosemary and additional bacon pieces as a garnish.

Twice Baked "potato" Zucchini

Cook Time: 45-50 minutes
Servings: 4

Ingredients:
- 2 zucchini squashes
- 4 strips bacon
- ½ cup shredded cheddar cheese
- ¼ cup minced onion
- ¼ cup sour cream
- 2 oz. cream cheese
- 2 tbsp melted butter
- 1 tbsp jalapeno pepper, minced
- Salt and pepper, to taste

Optional garnish:
- Jalapeno pepper slices, bacon crumbles

Method:
1. Preheat oven to 350 degrees (F) and retrieve a small ungreased baking dish.
2. Wash and dry the zucchini squash, and cut in half then long-wise (make 8 pieces). Use a spoon to scoop out the insides. Chop the scooped zucchini and put it in a bowl. Put the zucchini "boats" in the baking dish.
3. Add the other ingredients all in the bowl with the scooped zucchini and mash it all together until it is combined.
4. Divide the mixture evenly between the 8 pieces of zucchini and fill up the "boats". Then top with optional garnish.
5. Bake for 30 minutes or until the zucchini is tender and filled with bubbles.
6. Remove from oven and let them cool for 5 minutes before serving.

Snack

Roasted Garlic Spinach and Bacon Dip

Cook Time: approximately 1 hour
Servings: 6

Ingredients:
- 6 slices of bacon
- 5 oz. fresh spinach leaves
- 8 oz. softened cream cheese
- ½ cup sour cream
- 1 ½ tbsp fresh chopped parsley
- 1 tbsp roasted garlic
- Salt and pepper, to taste
- 1 tbsp lemon juice
- 2.5 oz. grated Parmesan cheese

Method:
1. Preheat oven to 350 degrees (F).
2. Cook the six slices of bacon on a skillet and until crisp. Remove bacon from skillet and place on a paper towel to drain off excess grease. Set aside.
3. Place the spinach in the bacon grease until it wilts down. Once it has wilted, set aside.
4. Add cream cheese, sour cream, parsley and roasted garlic to a bowl and mix together. Add salt and pepper to taste. Crumble bacon into the bowl and mix again.
5. Add the wilted spinach, some bacon grease, and lemon juice. Mix well.
6. Grate Parmesan cheese into the bowl and mix well again. Divide the mixture into three regular-sized ramekins.
7. Bake in the oven for 25 minutes, then broil for another 3 to 4 minutes or until browned on top.
8. Serve with pork rinds (optional) or use as a topping for other dishes.

Mini Cheesecakes

Cook Time: 35 minutes
Servings: 8

Ingredients:

Crust
- 2 tbsp butter
- ½ cup almond meal

Cheesecake
- 8 oz. of cream cheese
- 1 large egg
- ½ tsp vanilla extract
- ½ tsp lemon juice
- Pinch of salt
- ¼ cup erythritol or other sugar substitute

Method:

1. Preheat oven to 350 degrees F.
2. Make the crust by melting two tablespoons of butter and mix in the almond meal until it has the consistency of play dough.
3. Take about a teaspoon of the dough and press it into the bottom of a muffin tin. Repeat for the entire tin. You may want to use a cupcake liner to make it easy to remove the cheesecakes. Bake the crusts for about 5 minutes. They should be crispy and slightly brown.
4. Once the cream cheese reaches the room temperature, beat with rubber whisk until it is creamy. Once it gets creamy, add egg, vanilla extract, lemon, salt, and the sugar substitute. Beat it again until it is combined well.
5. Scoop the cream cheese mixture and place it over the baked crusts and fill the cups almost to the top.
6. Bake for 15 minutes. The cheesecake consistency should be a little jiggly. Let the cheesecakes cool in the fridge for 24 hours.
7. Once the cheesecakes are cool, slice and strawberries a dot of coconut butter for decoration (optional).

Freezer Fudge

We all get a sweet tooth now and then, or just need an extra treat. Here's a Keto freezer fudge recipe that is delicious and ready in just 20 minutes.

Cook Time: 30 minutes
Serves: 2-4

Ingredients:
- 1 cup coconut oil
- ¼ cup cocoa powder
- 8-10 drops of liquid stevia
- ½ to ¼ cup almond butter
- Pink salt or Maldon salt

Method:
1. Melt one cup of coconut oil.
2. Whisk in ¼ cup of cocoa powder and 8-10 drops of liquid stevia.
3. Add ¼ to ½ cup almond butter depending on the consistency preferred (if you are happy with coconut oil's thickness and texture, leave out the almond butter)
4. Fill an ice cube tray with the mixture.
5. Sprinkle a little pink salt or Maldon salt on top (this is optional).
6. Put the tray in the freezer – ready in just 20 minutes.

Zucchini Chips

Prepare for your next get-together or satisfy that longing for crunch with these tasty Tex-Mex style zucchini chips.

Cook Time: 25 minutes
Serves: 1

Ingredients:
- 1 large zucchini squash
- Salt
- 1 ½ cups coconut oil
- 1 tbsp Tex-Mex seasoning

Method:
1. Slice the zucchini squash into thin slices. Use a mandolin if possible.
2. Toss zucchini slices into a colander and sprinkle with salt. Let it sit for about 5 minutes, then press out excess water.
3. Heat coconut oil to 350 degrees (a fryer or a skillet).
4. Drop the zucchini slices into the oil and let them cook until they are golden brown. Then remove them and place on a paper towel.
5. Sprinkle squash with Tex-Mex or taco seasoning. Enjoy!

Other ideas: You can use a mixture of zucchini and yellow squash for more color. Dip the chips in salsa mix or sour cream for your preference.

Fat Bomb!

Cook Time: 15 minutes (after ingredients reach room temperature)
Serves: 2

Ingredients:
- 4.4 oz. (125g) cream cheese
- 4.4 oz. (125g) unsalted butter
- 2 tbsp cacao powder
- 1 tbsp sweetener (add more or less for preferred taste)

Method:
1. Allow cream cheese and unsalted butter to soften at room temperature.
2. Beat the cream cheese and butter with an rubber whisk for a minute, then add the cacao powder and sweetener in.
3. Beat mixture until it is smooth.
4. Place 1 to 2 teaspoons of mixture in mini baking cups and place in fridge until firm.

Coconut Berry Drops

Cook Time: About 20 minutes
Serves: 2

Ingredients:
- Cup coconut oil (refined)
- ½ cup frozen berries (raspberries, strawberries)
- 1 tsp vanilla extract
- 10-14 drops liquid stevia

Method:
1. Melt coconut oil in a pan. While it is melting, place frozen fruit in a processor to chop it into small pieces.
2. Add vanilla extract and stevia to the fruit. Then add melted coconut and process to mix it all together into a smooth blend. (If some berries are still frozen, warm them up in a pan over stovetop and put them back in for blending.)
3. Drop by spoonful of the mixture on parchment paper or scoop it into molds.
4. Place molds or parchment paper-lined container into the freezer to firm up the drops for about a half an hour. Store the remaining drops in a container in the freezer.

Lime Popsicles

Cook Time: 4 hours and 10 minutes
Servings: 6

Ingredients:
- 15 oz. can coconut milk
- ½ cup avocado (mashed)
- ½ cup fresh lime juice
- ¼ tsp vanilla stevia
- 1/8 tsp vanilla powder

Method:
1. Combine coconut milk, avocado, lime juice, vanilla stevia and powder in a blender or Vitamix. Blend all ingredients until it is a smooth consistency.
2. Spoon mixture into Popsicle molds and insert Popsicle sticks.
3. Freeze for 4 hours, then serve and enjoy!

Veggie Dip (A lot like hummus!)

Cook Time: 30 minutes
Servings: 6

Ingredients:
- 1 eggplant, sliced
- Pinch of salt
- 1 cup tahini
- 3-4 cloves of garlic
- 1-2 tbsp avocado oil
- 1 cup chopped parsley
- Salt and pepper, to taste

Method:
1. Slice the eggplant and lay slices out on a baking sheet that's lined with parchment paper. Salt the eggplant and allow it to sit for about 15 minutes. (This removes moisture)
2. Use a paper towel to pad dry excess water from the eggplant.
3. Broil eggplant for 5 to 8 minutes.
4. Remove skin if desired. (Leave it for the nutrients!)
5. Put eggplant in the food processor and pulse it for 3-5 minutes or until it's broken down.
6. Place the rest of the ingredients in the processor and blend on high until it is well combined and has a smooth consistency.
7. Serve with freshly chopped vegetables.

White chocolate Butter Pecan Fat Bomb

Cook Time: 20 minutes
Servings: 4

Ingredients:
- 2 tbsp coconut oil
- 2 oz. of cocoa butter
- 2 tbsp butter
- 2 tbsp erythritol (or another sweetener)
- 1 pinch of stevia
- 1 pinch of salt
- ¼ tsp vanilla extract
- ½ cup chopped pecans

Method:
1. Melt the coconut oil, cocoa butter, and butter in a small pan. Then turn the heat off.
2. Stir in the erythritol. Add the pinch of stevia and salt. Add the vanilla extract.
3. Add a few chopped pecans to the bottom of candy molds or cupcake molds. You can also choose to use hazelnuts, walnuts or macadamia nuts.
4. Pour the mixture into the molds on top of the nuts and place immediately in the freezer.
5. Let freeze for around 30 minutes.
6. Enjoy while they are nice and cool!

Chocolate Mousse

Cook Time: Less than 30 minutes
Servings: 8

Ingredients:
- 8 oz. of cream cheese
- ¼ cup unsweetened cocoa
- ½ avocado
- 2 to 3 tbsp of sweetener (stevia)
- 1/8 tsp vanilla extract
- ¼ cup heavy cream
- Shaved dark chocolate for garnish

Method:
1. Beat cream cheese with a handheld mixer until it is smooth and creamy. Slowly mix in cocoa, then add avocado and beat until smooth and creamy. (This might take about 5 minutes.)
2. Add sweetener and vanilla extract and beat one to two minutes until it is smooth.
3. In another bowl, whip the cream until it becomes stiff and forms peaks.
4. Place the whipped cream in with the cocoa mixture and fold together gently until it is all mixed.
5. Place mousse in a piping bag and fill containers. Use dark chocolate shavings as a garnish.

Keto Smoothie

Cook Time: 10 minutes
Serves: 1-2

Ingredients:
- 1 to 1 ¼ cup coconut milk (full fat)
- ½ avocado (frozen)
- 1 tbsp of nut butter (almond or macadamia)
- 1 tbsp chia seeds (presoaked in water for 10 minutes)
- 1 tbsp coconut oil
- Ice
- 2 tbsp cocoa
- Cacao nibs and cinnamon or optional toppings

Method:
1. Add all the contents into a blender and mix on high until smooth. Add a bit of water if needed to make a smooth consistency.
2. Top with cinnamon and cacao nibs.

Loaded Hassel back (not potatoes but) Zucchini

Cook Time: Less 30 minutes
Servings: 6

Ingredients:
- 3 zucchini squashes (medium sized)
- 6 to 8 oz. of your choice of cheese
- Salt and pepper, to taste
- 3 to 4 tbsp of sour cream
- 3 slices of bacon (cooked and crumbled)
- 2 to 3 tbsp chopped green onions

Method:
1. Preheat oven to 425 degrees (F).
2. Wash, dry and slice the ends off zucchini.
3. Slice zucchini squash by starting at one end and working toward the other – but without slicing all the way through. Try lining up chopsticks on either side of the squash and slice through until you hit the sticks.
4. Slice each of the zucchini squash in half to create 6 small Hassel backs.
5. Use foil to line a baking sheet, then arrange the squash on the sheet.
6. Stuff cheese between each of the discs. (Sliced cheese makes this step easiest.) Sprinkle with salt and pepper to taste.
7. Place another sheet of foil over the top and pinch the sides to form a pouch out of the foil. The pouch steams the squash and prevents the cheese from browning.
8. Bake in the oven for 15 to 20 minutes. Remove from oven and let it stand in the foil for another 5 minutes. Bake for 10 more minutes if you want them tenderer.
9. Once zucchini have reached the desired tenderness, top them off with the sour cream, bacon and onions.

Fast and Easy Blueberry Smoothie

Cook Time: 10 minutes
Servings: 2

Ingredients:

- 14 oz. coconut milk
- ½ cup blueberries (fresh or frozen)
- 1 tbsp fresh lemon juice
- ½ tsp vanilla extract

Method:

1. Put all the ingredients into a blender and mix on high until smooth. If you use canned coconut milk, it will make a creamier smoothie. Just remember to drain off the excess liquid.
2. Taste the smoothie and add more lemon juice for desired taste.

Mexican Chocolate Pudding

Cook Time: 10 minutes
Servings: 2

Ingredients:
- 1 avocado
- 2.5 tbsp raw cocoa powder
- 1 tbsp coconut milk
- ½ tsp pure vanilla extract
- 1 tbsp sweetener (coconut sugar, agave, or maple syrup)
- 1 tsp Ceylon cinnamon
- Pinch of stevia
- Pinch of cayenne pepper
- Pinch of pink Himalayan sea salt

Method:
1. Cut avocado, pit it, and blend the meat of it in a blender until it is smooth.
2. Add cocoa powder, coconut milk and vanilla extract and blend it together until smooth.
3. Add in your choice of sweetener, cinnamon, stevia and cayenne pepper.
4. Continue blending and scraping the sides of the processor to make sure there are no chunks. Blend it until it is smooth and well combined.
5. Serve pudding with a pinch of sea salt for flavor enhancement.

Conclusion

Achieving ketosis is not that difficult to do and it can have many health benefits. Are you ready to feel better and have more energy while losing weight? No matter what your health goals are, a Ketogenic diet can help you reach them. The good thing is, it's not difficult to do and you do not have to sacrifice taste to achieve it. In fact, you can get started with many of the simple recipes found here.

Use this book as a resource and refer back to it often. It can be a useful tool to assist you on your journey toward a healthier lifestyle. Try out the recipes, and maybe create a few of your own using Keto friendly ingredients. Thanks for reading – enjoy your journey!

Lightning Source UK Ltd.
Milton Keynes UK
UKHW050955100822
407113UK00007B/1527